Books should be returned or renewed by the
last date stamped above

SAVILL. A.

C152340079

The big book of Wheat-free Cooking

Awarded for excellence

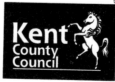

Kent
County
Council

The Big Book of
Wheat-Free Cooking

A fabulous collection of
180 seasonal recipes

Antoinette Savill

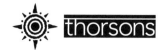

Thorsons
An Imprint of HarperCollins*Publishers*
77–85 Fulham Palace Road,
Hammersmith, London W6 8JB

The website address is: www.thorsonselement.com

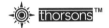

and *Thorsons* are trademarks of
HarperCollins*Publishers* Ltd

First published by Thorsons 2004

1 3 5 7 9 10 8 6 4 2

© 2004 Antoinette Savill

Contents

Acknowledgements

My thanks go to Wanda Whiteley, whose ideas and inspiration are invaluable and who has become a dear friend; to my mother Penny, who has so generously lent me her kitchen every time our house has become a building site and has selflessly helped test recipes in times of crisis; and to my stepfather Edward, who has relentlessly tasted at least 200 recipes! Lastly, my thanks to my husband Stephen, whose time-consuming help with my computer is inestimable.

How to Use the Symbols

The symbols shown below are used throughout the book to enable you to judge the suitability of each recipe. A wheat-free symbol is not included because *every* recipe is wheat free. An asterisk beside an ingredient indicates that it *may* contain gluten, so check and if necessary use an alternative gluten-free brand.

   Note that many of the recipes that are not marked as dairy free could be easily converted to such by using dairy-free margarine instead of butter and soya milk and yogurt in place of the standard dairy product. Similarly, many of the recipes that are not marked as vegetarian could easily be converted by using vegetarian products instead of meat – often you will find vegetarian options given in the introduction to the such recipes.

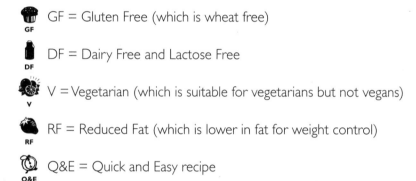

GF = Gluten Free (which is wheat free)

DF = Dairy Free and Lactose Free

V = Vegetarian (which is suitable for vegetarians but not vegans)

RF = Reduced Fat (which is lower in fat for weight control)

Q&E = Quick and Easy recipe

Becoming Wheat-Free

The buzzword for the future is wheat-watching. In countries such as the UK, Australia and the USA, the trend has already begun, with growing numbers of people avoiding wheat, either permanently or for short periods, to improve their health and energy.

However, when it comes to putting it into practice, the decision to go wheat free can be a little more difficult than one might think – not just because of the countless wheat-based products such as breads, pastas, pastries, cakes and cookies that are on the market but also because so many other products may surreptitiously contain wheat. You may be surprised to find that wheat is used to bulk out or stabilize many foods. For instance, nearly all processed, frozen or canned foods contain wheat, including soups, mayonnaise, sausages and frozen French fries. In addition, many manufactured products, such as soy sauce, contain very small amounts of wheat. Such tiny quantities may not cause problems for most people but those who have a wheat allergy or coeliac disease must ensure that everything they eat is entirely wheat free.

It's all too easy to dwell on the negative effects that some foods can have on us but we mustn't forget that food can act as a very healing medicine. It is vital then that we stop and consider what we are putting into our bodies and what effect it has on us physically and emotionally before we charge gung ho round the supermarket, throwing anything in our trolley.

Thankfully shopping has become a less arduous task for wheat-watchers over recent years, as an increasing number of wheat-free ingredients and products have become available. Take a look in the 'well-being' and organic aisles, for instance, and you'll find lots of interesting new wheat-free products from all over the world. Alternatively, you can buy the foods and ingredients that you need from health food shops, by mail order or on the internet (you'll find a helpful list of stockists on page 304).

Thanks to chefs like Jamie Oliver, cooking is now tremendously popular again – even amongst the young, many of whom are seeing it as cool for the first time. The TV food programs portray the fun and excitement of cooking and I want to show that cooking for food intolerance needn't be any different. The recipes in this book will ensure that cooking is an enjoyable experience – no matter what your age or level of experience.

With today's fast pace of life, shared family meals have inevitably become rare. Lifestyle changes and busy schedules mean that TV dinners and the general 'grab and graze' culture have become part of our way of looking at food and cooking it. However, I hope that the selection of quick, easy and comforting recipes in this book will encourage a return to everyone congregating in the kitchen and helping to prepare a delicious meal, as well as chatting and dining together.

My aim with this book is to provide plenty of delicious alternatives to products that normally contain wheat. You will therefore find the pages packed with wonderful breads, muffins, cakes, desserts and pies made with a wide variety of nutritious cereals such as rye, barley, oatmeal, rice, corn, millet and quinoa. And so that you can enjoy life to the full and not miss any of the normal foods that we eat on a day-to-day basis, I have also included many recipes that can be enjoyed by your family, your friends or at work – those who don't suffer from intolerances won't know the difference!

Improved health is the usual objective of those cutting out wheat – but it can have other advantages too. Wheat intolerance can be an important factor in a failure to shed excess weight. If you are eating a balanced diet and are in relatively good health yet still have difficulty losing weight, it may be that food intolerance is playing a part. This is because food intolerance can encourage the body to hold on to excess fluid. When the offending food is removed, weight loss often occurs. Abdominal bloating is often a sign that the digestive system is not dealing very well with a specific food and the most common food that is known to cause this problem is wheat.

The Trouble with Wheat

A large percentage of people eat too much wheat. If you think about the average daily diet, just three or four foods show up repeatedly. For example, an everyday breakfast of toast with butter and marmalade consists of wheat flour (bread), dairy (butter) and sugar (marmalade). A typical pasta salad for lunch would mean more wheat and dairy, whilst a dinner of pizza or chicken pie would again include wheat (in the pizza base or the pastry). And let's not forget snacks – biscuits, doughnuts, crispbreads and bagels are all popular snacks and each one contains wheat.

Many people don't think about the constituents of their meals and imagine they are eating lots of different foods. In fact, many meals are essentially the same but are processed, assembled or cooked differently.

Variety is the spice of life and one of the core principles of a healthy diet is exactly that – plenty of variety. If we eat a wheat-laden diet day in day out, year after year, it's no wonder our systems become overloaded, give up the struggle and become sluggish. Our bodies need the whole spectrum of nutrients and we cannot get these if we eat the same foods repeatedly.

Wheat has a nutritious and wholesome image because it is considered to be a good source of carbohydrates and dietary fibre. However, whilst we undoubtedly need both these elements in our diet, today's wheat flour is so over processed that the end product – the mass-produced bland bread that fills the supermarket shelves – bears little resemblance to the kind of healthy, wholemeal bread that our grandparents ate.

Since the arrival of mass production in the 1960s, wheat-filled foods have been the fastest growing items on the supermarket shelves. They are cheap and filling – which is what both the manufacturers and the majority of shoppers want – but, in order to produce the vast amounts of flour needed at the right price, wheat is sprayed with insecticides and fungicides. To then turn that wheat into bread can also involve an amazing number of processes. The wheat germ (which is high in vitamin E, has many of the B vitamins and is good for us) is often removed because it can turn rancid quickly and would therefore spoil the flour faster than the manufacturers would like. To make white flour, the bran is also removed; this is the outer part of the grain, which is a good source of niacin, iron, zinc, B vitamins and fibre. They may also irradiate the wheat in order to avoid contamination by insects. Having done all this, manufacturers then sometimes use chemicals, conditioners and preservatives to improve the texture and shelf life of the end product.

Unfortunately, all these processes result in most of the vitamins and minerals originally contained in the wheat being lost so the manufacturers often add synthetic vitamins and minerals, which the body has great difficulty absorbing.

Given this treatment, it's little wonder that the nutritional value of your average mass-produced loaf of wheat bread, or other wheat-laden products, is often rather poor. Personally, I would rather make my own – with the help of today's bread-making machines it's not the arduous task it once was.

Intolerances and Allergies

One of the main reasons that people give up wheat is because they discover – or suspect – that they have an intolerance to it. The exact cause of food intolerance is as yet unclear. However, repeated over-consumption of a particular food undoubtedly plays a central part in its development – hence the most common culprits in food intolerance are wheat, dairy produce, yeast and sugar.

Food intolerance can cause a myriad of symptoms and although they are usually mild at first, they often gradually worsen over the years. This list below outlines some of the most common symptoms of wheat intolerance:

- A bloated stomach
- Regular flatulence (gas) or indigestion
- Diarrhoea or constipation for no apparent reason
- Fluid retention
- Grogginess on waking in the morning
- Feeling permanently tired
- Brain fog or sleepiness after eating a wheat-filled snack or meal
- Headaches

- Aches and pains for no apparent reason
- Skin conditions
- A craving for foods containing wheat
- Fluctuating weight despite having a very healthy diet, exercising regularly and drinking plenty of water

Food intolerance is notoriously difficult to detect because the reaction to the offending food is slow and symptoms are not felt for a few days. It is therefore not easy to connect the offending food to the symptoms it causes. Also, given that the culprit food is usually one that we eat very regularly, the symptoms can be on-going and we often attribute them to something completely different, such as stress. There are certain conditions that are now strongly linked to food intolerance; in particular an intolerance to wheat or dairy. Irritable bowel syndrome (IBS) is a prime example – when wheat is removed from the diet the condition often improves dramatically or clears up completely.

There are various tests available for food intolerance, though generally these should be treated with caution, as many of them are unreliable. Your doctor will be able to arrange for you to see a qualified nutritionist who can oversee accurate tests for food intolerance but this is not a service provided on the NHS in the UK and it can be expensive. The only alternative is to eliminate the suspect food from your diet completely for a period of five weeks and monitor the results. If, on reintroducing the food, your symptoms reoccur then this will prove your guess was correct. However, please make sure that you always consult your doctor, as some symptoms can be indicative of a medical problem.

If you suffer from many of the symptoms outlined on page 3 after eating wheat then you should notice a huge difference if you avoid it for about a month. You should feel energized and clear-headed, rather than exhausted and under par. Do be aware, though, that one of the quirks of food intolerance is that sufferers often crave the offending food and can experience withdrawal symptoms for a short period when the particular food is removed from the diet. However, these symptoms usually pass relatively quickly.

The good news is that food intolerance, unlike food allergy, is not for life. By avoiding the culprit food for a period, most people find that they can tolerate it occasionally, although problems will generally resurface if it is eaten on a regular basis. Unadulterated organic wheat flour or Spelt can sometimes be eaten by people with mild wheat intolerance – because all the original goodness and fibre is still there – but I have not used these ingredients in the recipes as this does not apply to everyone and such breads and pastas can be purchased from good health food shops.

There is a real difference between food intolerance and food allergy: Whereas an intolerance causes delayed symptoms, an allergy usually produces an immediate and often extreme physical reaction to the offending substance or food. This is a result of the speed of the immune system's reaction to the allergen. In some instances the response can be so severe that it results in anaphylactic shock. Thankfully, despite the publicity given to such cases, they are rare and food allergy itself is far more rare than food intolerance. Those with a severe wheat *allergy* should look out for the * symbol in the recipe, as this indicates a product that may contain a very small amount of gluten – and the source of that gluten could be wheat.

Unfortunately allergies are very often life-long, as is coeliac disease. In this serious condition, the lining of the colon wall is affected by gluten (found in certain grains such as rye, barley and oats), which causes malabsorption of nutrients, severe pain and symptoms such as diarrhoea. (As mentioned above, any ingredient that could contain gluten is marked with an asterisk and coeliacs should ensure the product they use is gluten free.) The test for coeliac disease is a straightforward one but there are certain people who, although they have tested negative, still find they feel much better if they eliminate gluten from their diet.

Some Practical Pointers

Becoming wheat free does require a bit of forethought but this will ensure your diet is both effective *and* enjoyable. There is no point getting better but feeling deprived and miserable! A little organization will help you have a varied and interesting diet that won't leave you feeling that you're missing out. The following tips should help make the transition to a wheat-free diet as smooth as possible.

- Make a list of the normal foods that you would eat over a couple of days and buy wheat-free alternatives. If you usually have a wheat cereal for breakfast then put wheat-free cereals on your shopping list – for example, gluten-free muesli, porridge oats, cornflakes and rice pops – or if you have toast, add wheat-free breads to your list.
- If you work in an office, take time to plan your lunch as it will not be easy to buy wheat-free sandwiches. I suggest making up your own delicious lunch box – it will probably be cheaper and less hassle than eating out anyway. You can make up your choice of wheat-free sandwiches or rolls – why not try out some new flavours such as smoked trout and avocado or chicken tikka and roasted red peppers.
- When you cook, think about making extra portions. For instance, if you are cooking on Sunday make an extra portion so that you can take some into work for lunch on Monday. Equally, if you are having a night in, make a big pan of soup and save some to take into lunch over a couple of days. And don't forget to keep a stock of emergency rations if you have a sweet tooth. Ready-made cookies or cakes are great for convenience or you can make your own cakes or muffins at the weekend and take them to work over the following days. Some recipes in this book last the whole week, such as the fruit, chocolate or ginger cake.
- Dinner is of course much easier than some other meals, but it is still important to plan ahead. The last thing you want is to be so hungry that you grab the first thing you can find – which will probably have wheat in it. If you live alone or with a partner who doesn't mind going wheat free, it's a good idea to go through your cupboards, refrigerator and deep-freeze and throw out any products containing wheat. If you have a family to feed then it helps to put all the wheat products in one cupboard or one part of the refrigerator/freezer

and keep a wheat-free zone for yourself. However, the recipes in this book are designed to be eaten by the whole family – they're so delicious that no one will notice they're wheat free.

- If you are at home with tiny tots and toddlers ensure you are not hungry when you are feeding them, as it is very difficult not to be tempted into nibbling at their food, and fish fingers or cakes, chicken nuggets, sausages – not to mention cookies, cakes or sandwiches – are all full of wheat. If you are going to a children's party where all the other parents will be tucking in to birthday cake and pastries, take your own special treats so that you can relax and have fun.
- When you start wheat-watching you are going to have to get used to reading the label on every product that you buy. It is pretty time consuming and boring but you will be surprised by how many foods contain wheat. Try to remember a few of these products and brands each time you shop and the process will soon get quicker.
- It is worth taking some wheat-free supplies with you when you go on holiday. Some hotels will cater for certain diets but they are unlikely to provide all the products you would like. You will be much more relaxed if you take your own crispbreads, oatcakes, sliced bread, snacks and so on.
- Use the wide range of resources that are now available to those with intolerances. Because of the increased demand in many countries, plenty of new wheat-free food ranges are now being produced and much more information about food intolerances and allergies is available from medical and alternative practitioners. The Internet also has lots of useful information and a wide selection of recipes from all over the world to help and guide people who wish to become wheat free.

Many people who initially see a wheat-free diet as restrictive soon come to view it as a form of liberation. Often people eat a lot of wheat because it has become a habit and it is convenient. However, when wheat is restricted it opens people's eyes to the wide variety of foods that they are missing out on. By necessity, people begin to prepare a wider variety of foods and most find that they enjoy this healthy way of eating so much that they continue to eat this way indefinitely, and have just the occasional wheat product.

Be Sensible

If you are intolerant to wheat, it is important not to become obsessive about the whole thing. Yes in a perfect world we would avoid wheat entirely (and of course you must do if you are allergic to wheat or are a coeliac) but why go to extremes when it is unnecessary? As we know, many manufactured products do contain very small amounts of wheat but if you eat these products only occasionally you should not have an adverse reaction. Soy sauce is a good example. Ordinary soy sauce contains a very small amount of wheat and is therefore unlikely to cause any problems for someone who eats the odd meal cooked with it. Wheat-free soy sauce is available in the shops but if you convince yourself that you must only have the wheat-free brand then you'll worry every time you eat out at a Chinese restaurant – which defeats the point of going out.

Make sensible choices when eating out; there will always be an alternative to wheat-based meals. An Italian restaurant, for example, will have much more than pasta and pizza – try risotto or fish. Alternatively, you can ask them to cook some dishes to suit you – cooking escallops without the flour and breadcrumbs, for instance, perhaps with some tomato sauce or with some sage and lemon juice, would not be too much trouble and chefs are generally very obliging.

Choose simple food that is more likely to be wheat free, such as salads to start or fruit and Parma ham followed by steamed or roast fish, vegetables and grilled meats. Avoid all the pastries, soufflés and hot puddings and instead have delicious sorbets, ice creams, fruit poached in liqueur, fresh fruit salad or a wicked chocolate or fruit mousse. Do not be tempted by petits fours with coffee, but do enjoy top quality or hand-made chocolates.

Enjoy Your Food

Your social life does not need to stop because you are following a wheat-free diet. Have fun trying out new recipes and make life easy for yourself by putting together quick and easy ideas with something a bit more complicated – never (unless you have all the time in the world) combine three really advanced recipes in one evening or you will be exhausted and past enjoying yourself by the time dinner is served!

With all cooking, you need to enjoy tasting the food at the beginning, in the middle and at the end. Season with your fingers and not with a spoon so that you are in touch with your food. If you are cooking without wheat and dairy you will probably need more seasoning and the magic of fresh herbs or spices to perk up the food. Dried herbs and spices lose their flavour very quickly so buy small amounts frequently rather than a large amount, which will soon loose its essential flavour. With practice, it will soon be easy to judge how much extra seasoning you need to make your food perfect for your palate

A varied diet is a healthy and exciting one so be adventurous and try wheat-free recipes from around the globe – Chinese, Thai, Vietnamese, Japanese, Malaysian or Indonesian dishes will seldom contain wheat as they usually use rice instead. However, avoid wheat noodles and anything dipped in batter. Indian food is generally great for cooking at home or for takeaways as they usually use gram flour for poppadums and most of the dishes are served with rice and thickened with yogurt. Avoid naan and other breads, and vegetables dipped in batter, and you should be fine. Some Mexican recipes, like tortillas, tacos and nachos, are usually made with corn and are delicious with chilli sauce, guacamole, and spicy meats. There is a delicious recipe for wraps in this book, which you can use with all sorts of alternative fillings, such as chicken tikka, slices of roast tuna and sweet red peppers, cold roast beef and guacamole, to name just a few.

Be Flexible

Wheat-free flours play an important part in many of the recipes in this book so I suggest that you stock up on different kinds. There is nothing worse than finding you have run out – particularly when it can require a major trip or an internet order for you to replenish supplies. You'll be disappointed you cannot make that cake or pastry and, in my experience, it's tempting to using a bit of leftover wheat flour – which would, of course, ruin your efforts to be wheat free.

These days, our busy lifestyles mean we need to have a flexible approach to food. This is reflected in these recipes, which can be adapted to suit your tastes and needs. It is easy, for instance, to halve or double the quantities according to your needs. You can also play around with the ingredients. If you like the general idea of the recipe but not the main ingredient you can, for example, swap salmon for a similar oily fish such as tuna, marlin or swordfish. A turkey recipe, for example, can be swapped with chicken, pheasant or guinea fowl. Red meats can be changed to other red meats and so on. You can substitute fresh or dried fruits with different varieties and combinations and substitute dairy products with goat, sheep or alternative dairy-free products. In my view, a good recipe book should provide ideas and inspiration and should be followed in a relaxed and enjoyable way.

Think Local and Organic

One of the aims of this book is to show you how easy it is to convert to the wheat-free way of eating so that you can feel confident enough to try all sorts of delicious foods. There is no danger of becoming bored with these new recipes – they're fun, easy to prepare, interesting, delicious and, with a little help from you, they'll be forever evolving.

I have selected many seasonal recipes, as I believe in eating food that is grown or reared in this country and which is sold in season. I am not a great fan of foods being flown from all around the world, picked too early and sold unripe. I am, however, a great fan of organic foods, farmers' markets and local produce. With organic produce, the difference in taste – aside from the lack of chemicals and preservatives – is enough to convince me that the extra effort is worthwhile. Why not try some of the recipes using only organic products and see if you think there is a marked difference in sweetness, flavour and texture?

If you only buy a dozen organic products each week, I would always recommend that you opt for organic dairy products, eggs, chicken, tomatoes and carrots, as these make the biggest difference to the recipes.

I have always loved cooking and entertaining at home; my boundless enthusiasm for excellent food is equalled by my fascination for creating new and contemporary allergy-free recipes for all occasions throughout the year. Warm and comforting food in winter, and cool and refreshing dishes in summer all add up to a diverse and exciting food year. I hope my desire to make cooking without wheat rewarding and fun is reflected in my recipes and that you will have hours of pleasure preparing and enjoying them.

At-a-Glance Do's and Don'ts for a Healthy, Wheat-Free Diet

Do: Drink 1.5 litres/1½ quarts of pure still water each day, but not during main meals

Don't: Get so hungry that you eat anything

Do: Keep wheat-free emergency snacks like hummus, guacamole, crispbreads, nachos, bread rolls and cookies in the refrigerator or store cupboard

Don't: Bolt your food, even if it is wheat-free this will not help your digestion

Do: Use leftover titbits of wheat-free pastry to make little tarts, for example leftover vegetables and cheese or jam (jelly) and fruit

Don't: Continue to use the same set of wooden spoons if you are changing your diet to gluten, wheat- or dairy-free – buy some new ones

Do: Freeze leftover wheat-free bread as breadcrumbs for bread sauce, toppings or stuffing

Don't: Forget to clean out your store cupboard, refrigerator and deep-freeze of products containing wheat

Do: Buy a bread maker and ice cream maker if possible

Don't: Use your bread maker for wheat bread as it will contaminate your loaf

Do: Scrupulously wash out your baking tins, bowls and containers before using for wheat-free cooking if you have used them for recipes that include wheat

Don't: Forget to stock up on different types of wheat-free flours for all your recipes

Do: Make shopping lists and allow extra time in the shops for reading the labels

Don't: Panic buy, instead plan your meals, office or school lunch box and entertaining in advance

At-a-Glance Guide to Common Foods That Contain Wheat, Gluten and Dairy

These lists are very basic so please do always read the labels before purchasing any products; the most surprising foods contain wheat, gluten or dairy.

Foods Containing Wheat

Watch out for:

WHEAT PROTEIN, BINDER, THICKENER OR THICKENING

PITTA BREADS AND WRAPS, CHAPATTI AND NAAN BREAD

TORTILLAS, NACHOS CHIPS WITH A MIX OF WHEAT AND CORN

YORKSHIRE PUDDINGS, PANCAKES, WAFFLES, TOAD IN THE HOLE

BATTER-COATED FISH OR VEGETABLES

NOODLES, POT NOODLES, PASTA, GNOCCHI

CAKES, COOKIES, PASTRIES, SCONES, MUFFINS, DOUGHNUTS

BREADS, BREADSTICKS

BREADCRUMBS IN STUFFING; CRUMB-COATED FISH, CHICKEN OR VEGETABLES

RUSK IN SAUSAGES, BURGERS AND OTHER MEAT PRODUCTS

PIES, SAUSAGE ROLLS AND SPRING ROLLS

SOME CHOCOLATES AND CHOCOLATE BARS, OTHER SWEETS AND CANDIES

ALL PREPARED CHILLER CABINET FOODS AND SAUCES

ALL READY-MADE FROZEN MEALS, SNACKS AND DISHES

MOST CANNED PREPARED FOODS, SAUCES AND SOUPS

DURUM WHEAT (PASTA FLOUR) AND SPELT (FLOUR)

SEMOLINA, COUSCOUS AND KIBBLED WHEAT

BOUILLON OR STOCK CUBES

MOST BREAKFAST CEREALS AND INSTANT OATMEAL PREPARATIONS

MOST CRISPBREADS, CHEESE BISCUITS AND COCKTAIL BISCUITS (TWIGLETS ETC.) AND
  CANAPÉS

CRUMBLE MIX AND CAKE, MUFFIN, BROWNIE AND COOKIE MIXES

CAULIFLOWER AND MACARONI CHEESE AND WELSH RAREBIT

CAESAR SALAD WITH CROÛTONS AND ANY CROÛTONS WITH SOUPS

CROISSANTS, BRIOCHE AND GARLIC BREAD

CUSTARD POWDER AND SAUCE

DUMPLINGS AND DANISH PASTRIES

QUICHES AND TARTS

SCOTCH EGGS

STEAMED PUDDINGS, SCONES AND CRUMPETS

SLICED PROCESSED HAM, TURKEY AND MEATS

MOST VEGETARIAN PREPARED DISHES

SOME PÂTÉS AND MOST MOUSSES

Foods Containing Gluten

Watch out for:

RYE, BARLEY, OATS, BRAN

MALTED PRODUCTS, MALT VINEGAR, MALT, MALT WHISKY

STARCH (INCLUDING MODIFIED STARCH)

MIXED SPICE (PIE SPICE) AND OTHER BLENDED SEASONINGS

ALL OF THE FOODS PREVIOUSLY LISTED AS CONTAINING WHEAT

Foods Containing Dairy

Watch out for:

BUTTER, BUTTERMILK, MARGARINE OR SHORTENING CONTAINING WHEY

MILKSHAKES, MILK SOLIDS, SKIMMED MILK POWDER, NON-MILK FAT SOLIDS

HARD CHEESE, SOFT CHEESE AND CHEESE DIPS

YOGURT, ICE CREAMS AND FROZEN DESSERTS

HYDROLYSED WHEY PROTEIN, LACTOSE, LACTIC ACID, CASEIN

BATTER AND CAKE OR COOKIE MIXES

HOT CHOCOLATE MIXES, CONDENSED OR EVAPORATED MILK

CREAM, CRÈME FRAÎCHE AND FROMAGE FRAIS

CUSTARDS, SWEET AND SAVOURY SAUCES

MASHED POTATO-TOPPED DISHES

CAKE TOPPINGS

RICE PUDDING AND INSTANT MIXES

ALL PREPARED CHILLER CABINET FOODS

ALL FROZEN PREPARED FOODS

MOST CANNED FOODS, SAUCES AND SOUPS

The Big Book of Wheat-Free Cooking

CHOCOLATES AND SWEETS

MOST CAKES, PASTRIES, COOKIES AND BREADS

SOME SLICED TURKEY, HAM AND OTHER MEAT PREPARATIONS

SOME PÂTÉS AND ALL MOUSSES

My List of Useful Ingredients

My store cupboard positively groans with food and drink so that I never run short of anything wheat free. Here is a short list of the most useful ingredients and foods that you might like to have in your store cupboard, refrigerator or deep-freeze. As well as wheat-free products, I have included some gluten- and dairy-free suggestions, which may be helpful for coeliacs and those on combined diets. If you can buy organic produce and products whenever possible you will notice a great difference in the taste, texture and quality of the finished recipe.

In the Store Cupboard

Antoinette Savill gluten-free white loaf, bread rolls and pizza bases

Prepared gluten- and wheat-free flour mixes such as Wellfoods, Doves Farm or Orgran

Doves Farm rice, buckwheat, organic rye, or other organic brands of barley, millet, oat, corn flours (these can be mixed or used individually according to the recipe)

Quinoa, amaranth, millet flakes for muesli

Nature's Path Mesa Sunrise (multi-grain breakfast cereal)

Gluten-free baking powder, bicarbonate of soda (baking soda), cream of tartar and cornflour (cornstarch)

Organic instant polenta and organic ready-made blocks of polenta

Unrefined granulated and golden caster (superfine) sugar, unrefined soft light brown and soft dark brown sugar and icing (confectioners') sugar

Organic ground almonds, walnuts, Brazil nuts, pine nuts and whole almonds

Organic sunflower, pumpkin and sesame seeds

Doves Farm organic gluten-free Lemon Zest Cookies

Cold pressed organic honey, black strap molasses, treacle, golden (corn) syrup

Cherry, raspberry and apricot jams (jellies) and marmalade

Pure Madagascan vanilla extract and Boyajian pure citrus oils (lime, lemon and orange for icing cakes)

Gluten- or wheat-free fast-acting or instant yeast

Wheat- and/or dairy-free chocolate with at least 72% cocoa solids such as Green & Black's organic or 73% El Rey

Cold pressed extra virgin olive oil, avocado oil and pumpkin oil

Organic balsamic vinegar, cider vinegar, unsweetened carrot juice

Wheat-free tomato sauce and purée (paste)

Ground spices and fresh ginger and chilli

Dried herbs and fresh herbs and garlic

Canned clear consommé (beef and chicken) and a packet of gelatine

Chopped chillies in oil; soy sauce and Worcestershire sauce

Wild, brown and risotto rice

Orgran wheat-, gluten-, yeast-free pasta shapes, spaghetti, lasagne and fettuccini

Canned organic chickpeas (garbanzos), puy lentils and cannellini beans

Canned reduced-fat coconut milk and cartons of coconut cream

Canned chopped tomatoes, white crab meat and anchovies

Provamel Alpro dairy-free long life organic unsweetened soya and vanilla milk

Provamel Alpro dairy-free chocolate and caramel desserts, organic Yofu yogurts

and Soya Dream (substitute cream)

In the Refrigerator

Apart from all the usual fresh foods in the refrigerator, I keep the following essentials for my recipes:

Provamel Alpro Soya Chilled (the best fresh dairy-free milk)

Elmlea single, whipping and double cream or organic dairy creams if preferred

Organic or half-fat crème fraîche, reduced-fat Philadelphia cream cheese

Sunblush tomatoes, pitted black and green olives in oil

Fresh pesto and fresh tomato salsa (from pasta or deli sections in stores)

Large and medium-sized organic free-range eggs

Organic butter, dairy-free hard margarine, organic Pure soft margarine

Buttermilk, lard and vegetable shortening (Trex or Cookeen are both good)

Dairy-free Tofutti mozzarella-style cheese slices, Sour Supreme sour cream substitute and three flavours of Creamy Smooth soft cream-style cheese

Dairy-free Redwood Wholefood Company Cheezly dairy-free Feta style cheese in oil and grated Cheddar-style cheese

A selection of wheat-free mustards

In the Deep-freeze

I try not to keep much in the deep-freeze because I prefer fresh food but for convenience and emergencies, I have the following:

Organic chicken breasts
Streaky and smoked back bacon
Organic frozen vegetables
Salmon steaks, large tiger prawns (jumbo shrimp), crayfish tails and smoked salmon
Gluten- or wheat-free sausages (Sainsbury's Toulouse sausages are excellent)
Tofutti dairy-free ice creams to serve with puddings or Baked Alaska
The Village Bakery organic wheat- or gluten-free Chocolate Almond Cake, Lemon Cake and
    Baltic Rye and Raisin Borodinsky Rye

Introduction to the Recipes

With this cookbook, I have tried to balance the number of quick and easy recipes with those that are more time consuming. This should appeal not only to working people with very limited time for entertaining, but also to those juggling a demanding family life. Hopefully, even people who don't like cooking will enjoy the quick and easy recipes, which I have marked with a Q&E symbol.

I have used various different types or blends of flour in the recipes; some, like Orgran self-raising, are very light, while others, such as rye, are very heavy. This means that if you are using American cup measures and substitute a different flour for that given in the recipe you may need to use your own judgement as to how much to use.

There is a wide range of gluten and wheat-free flour available. My favourite, and the one that I use in many of the recipes, is made by Wellfoods Ltd and is a particularly good mix. It can be purchased by mail order (see page 304 for information) but is not available in the shops yet. Two very good flours that are available in the shops are Doves Farm gluten-free flour and Orgran self-raising flour. You can, of course, mix your own blend to suit but don't use just one kind of flour, instead mix something like rice flour with potato flour and barley or corn flour (cornstarch), depending on your dietary needs. Please take into consideration that each variety of flour has a different absorbency level and quantities of flour and liquid must therefore be adjusted accordingly. Sometimes you may need to add a little extra liquid if the mixture is too stiff or dry; alternatively, if the mixture is too wet, you may need to add a fraction more flour. If you keep using the same brands or mix of flour, you will soon be able to judge this without a moment's thought.

In order to balance out the more indulgent and calorific recipes, I have included a substantial number of reduced-fat recipes. Some of them may seem very easy and incredibly healthy but I feel that it is important that in our excitement at being able to bake and cook unlimited delicious meals, we don't forget the need to have some meals that aid our digestion and that are packed full of nutrients.

In response to the many emails I have received over the past few years, I have tried to incorporate some special requests. For the first time in any of my cookbooks I have indicated when a recipe is suitable for freezing. I have also written a selection of seasonal menus for those of you who find this useful, with some hints on how best to create your own perfectly balanced menus (see pages 291–297). Thank you to all those who sent emails – it's great to hear how much my books help.

Throughout the book, all solid and liquid ingredients are given in metric first followed by American imperial and cup measurements. Please follow one set of measurements in each recipe, as they are not interchangeable. All recipes have been tested using each set of measurements.

Please note that where a recipe involves using any specific size of baking tin (pan) or anything other than basic kitchen equipment, this is listed below the ingredients – hopefully this should prevent anyone from beginning a recipe only to discover they don't have the necessary equipment.

Unless otherwise stated all tablespoon or teaspoon measures are level. All eggs are medium unless otherwise stated. As I think that it makes a substantial difference to the colour, texture and taste of the recipes, I always use organic eggs and chicken. All dairy products are also specified as organic. This is because after a long period of abstaining from dairy, some people – myself included – can tolerate organic dairy products. I believe that this is because chemicals, additives, preservatives, antibiotics and pesticides are not present and hence the body finds it easier to digest the product. Organic products in general have been used in all the recipes but I leave the choice of whether or not you use them to your discretion. A number of the recipes specify particular gluten-free ingredients – these can be purchased in large supermarkets or superstores, health food shops or by mail order.

Before you start a recipe, please look through it carefully and ensure that anyone who may eat it does not have an intolerance to any of the ingredients. It would be so annoying and such a waste of time and money to prepare a dish that one person could not eat!

You will find the recipes organized into groups, usually according to their main ingredient. Where recipes are categorized by the circumstances in which they are usually served, for instance as an appetizer or a breakfast dish, do not feel bound by this – use recipes how you want to use them. An appetizer, for example, can be served as a main course for fewer people, while a breakfast muffin can be a great snack at any time of the day.

I hope these little snippets of information help make wheat-watching easy as well as rewarding.

Soups ...

Leek and Rocket Soup

For a simple and filling lunch, serve this delicious soup with just a hunk of Rye and Barley Soda Bread* or Walnut Bread* (pages 271 and 273). For dinner parties you can serve it with Mini Rosemary and Orange Muffins (see page 275), a flourish of extra crème fraîche or Soya Dream and a single rocket (arugula) leaf for decoration.

GF	DF	V	RF	Q&E

Serves 4

500g/1lb 2oz packet extra-trimmed leeks, ends trimmed and discarded

55g/2oz organic butter or dairy-free margarine

500ml/2 cups warm allergy-free vegetable stock (bouillon)

55g/2oz packet prepared rocket (arugula) leaves, keep 4 leaves back for decoration

125ml/½ cup half-fat crème fraîche or Provamel dairy-free Soya Dream

200ml/¾ cup organic semi-skimmed milk or organic unsweetened dairy-free soya milk

Sea salt and freshly ground black pepper

Optional

Extra half-fat crème fraîche or dairy-free Soya Dream for decoration

* coeliacs please use gluten-free alternatives

Slice the leeks very thinly and rinse under cold running water. Melt the butter or margarine in a pan over low heat, add the leeks and gently cook until soft. Stir from time to time but make sure the leeks keep their bright colour.

Put the hot leeks, the stock (bouillon), rocket (arugula) and crème fraîche or Soya Dream into a blender and blend until smooth. Pour the soup back into the pan, add the milk and seasoning and simmer over low heat until hot.

Fennel and Parsnip Soup

This soup has a subtle aniseed flavour that is imparted by the fennel. You can serve it with the Olive and Rosemary Bread* on page 274 or the Walnut Bread* on page 273.

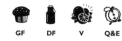

GF **DF** **V** **Q&E**

Serves 6–8

55g/2oz organic butter or dairy-free margarine
1 large onion, finely chopped
455g/1lb parsnips, peeled and chopped
340g/12oz fennel bulb, finely diced
Sea salt and freshly ground black pepper
1 tablespoon wheat-free flour mix*
1 teaspoon curry powder* or curry paste*
1 litre/4 cups hot allergy-free vegetable stock (bouillon)
125ml/½ cup organic milk or organic unsweetened dairy-free soya milk
125ml/½ cup organic cream or dairy-free Provamel Soya Dream

Optional
Chopped parsley or chives for decoration

* coeliacs please use gluten-free ingredients

Melt the butter or margarine in a pan over low heat, add the onion, parsnips, fennel, salt and pepper and cook gently until softened but not browned. Stir in the flour and curry powder or paste and gradually incorporate the hot stock (bouillon).

Simmer the vegetables until they are soft. Allow them to cool then place in a blender and blend until smooth.

Return the soup to the pan, stir in the milk, cream or Soya Dream, adjust the seasoning and heat through. Sprinkle with some parsley or chives and serve.

Carrot and Swede Soup

This soup has a very subtle combination that most people cannot quite put their finger on. You can serve the soup with the Mini Rosemary and Orange Muffins on page 275.

GF   DF   V   RF   Q&E

Serves 8

4 tablespoons cold pressed extra virgin olive oil
455g/1lb organic carrots, peeled and chopped
565g/1lb 4oz swede, peeled and chopped
3 celery sticks, tough strings removed, chopped
1 red onion, finely sliced
2 litres/8 cups hot allergy-free vegetable stock (bouillon)
Salt and freshly ground black pepper

Optional
Half-fat crème fraîche or dairy-free Soya Dream to decorate and a little chopped fresh parsley

Warm the oil in a big pan, add all the vegetables and cook gently over medium heat until softened. Stir in the stock (bouillon) and simmer for about 25 minutes. Allow the vegetables and liquid to cool then place in a blender and blend until smooth.

Return the soup to the pan and season to taste. Reheat the soup, pour into serving bowls and decorate with a teaspoon of crème fraîche or dairy-free Soya Dream and chopped parsley.

Cauliflower and Roquefort Soup

This soup is pale, subtle and sophisticated and complements a main course of red meat or game. You can of course use any kind of leftover cheese for informal occasions.

GF   V   Q&E

Serves 4

55g/2oz organic butter
1 large onion, finely chopped
1 small cauliflower, trimmed and cut into florets
½ tablespoon allergy-free vegetable bouillon powder
1 litre/4 cups boiling filtered water
115g/4oz organic Roquefort cheese, crumbled (do not use a strong cheese)
125ml/½ cup organic cream
Sea salt and freshly ground black pepper
1 tablespoon chopped fresh chives

Melt the butter in a pan over moderate heat, add the onions and cook until soft. Add the cauliflower and cook for 5 minutes, stirring frequently so that the vegetables don't brown. Add the bouillon powder and the hot water and simmer at bubbling point for about 20 minutes.

Cool slightly before blending with the crumbled cheese and cream. Return to the pan and season with salt and pepper. Serve piping hot with a sprinkling of chives.

Onion Soup with Goats' Cheese Croûtons

French onion soup is my favourite soup and it is often served with hard cheese melted on slices of French bread or a poached egg and grated cheese. Here is a similar idea that is equally delicious and very easy to make.

Serves 4

GF　　V　　Q&E

30g/1oz organic butter

2 tablespoons cold pressed extra virgin olive oil

3 large red onions, sliced very finely

2 garlic cloves, crushed

2 teaspoons balsamic vinegar

1 litre/4 cups allergy-free beef stock (bouillon) or use consommé and water mixed

Sea salt and freshly ground black pepper

Freshly grated nutmeg

4 very thick slices gluten-free white bread (see page 304 for stockist), crusts removed

2 × 100g/3½oz packets Capricorn or any other medium-soft round goats' cheese with a rind, each one sliced in half horizontally

---

Heat the butter with the oil in a large pan, add the onions and cook over a low heat until softened. Stir in the garlic and cook for another couple of minutes. Stir in the balsamic vinegar and cook for a few more minutes. Pour in the stock (bouillon) or consommé and water mix and season with salt, pepper and nutmeg.

Simmer the soup for about 35 minutes until the onions are soft and the soup has reduced slightly.

Using a round metal pastry cutter, stamp a large enough circle out of each slice of bread to enable you to place one slice of goats' cheese on top. Grill (broil) one side of each slice of bread until dark golden, turn over and top with the goats' cheese and a little black pepper. Grill (broil) them until golden and melting but not collapsed.

Ladle the soup into warm bowls and top with the goats' cheese croûtons.

Chilled Avocado Soup

This soup really does need to be chilled and served within 2 hours, so that the amazing colour remains bright. It's lucky that it is so quick and easy to prepare!

Serves 2 as a main course, or 3 as an appetizer

GF   DF   V   Q&E

Stock (bouillon)
425ml/1¾ cups allergy-free vegetable stock (bouillon) or boiling water flavoured with 2 teaspoons of allergy-free vegetable bouillon powder

Salsa
¼ small red onion, finely chopped

¼ red pepper and ¼ yellow pepper (bell pepper), seeded and finely chopped

2 heaped tablespoons coarsely chopped coriander (cilantro) leaves

7.5cm/3in cucumber, peeled and finely chopped

1 tablespoon cold pressed extra virgin olive oil

2 teaspoons lemon juice

Soup
2 large ripe avocados, halved, stoned (pitted) and all the flesh scraped out

2 tablespoons lemon juice

Chilli sauce*, paste* or chillies minced in oil

Sea salt and freshly ground black pepper

* coeliacs please use gluten-free ingredients

First, make the vegetable stock (bouillon) and allow it to become cold.

Make the salsa: mix the ingredients in the given order in a small bowl and toss until evenly mixed. Cover and chill until ready to serve the soup.

Now make the soup: put the avocado flesh into a blender, pour in the cold stock (bouillon) and blend until smooth. Pour the soup into a bowl; adjust the seasoning with the lemon juice, chilli, salt and pepper. Cover and chill. I usually put it in the deep-freeze for 30 minutes.

Divide the soup between the soup dishes and decorate with plenty of salsa. Serve immediately.

Pumpkin Soup with Creole Seeds

I spent six months in the Hamptons, Long Island, some years ago and one of my favourite scenes was the pumpkin field in full bloom. I had never cooked a pumpkin before and was amazed at the variety of colours and sizes. Since then, every autumn (fall), I have enjoyed making this soup and a pumpkin pie for Halloween, just as I did years ago. This soup freezes well.

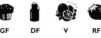

Serves 6

GF   DF   V   RF

1 large onion, finely chopped
2 tablespoons cold pressed extra virgin olive oil
2 garlic cloves, crushed
1 teaspoon cumin seeds
1 heaped teaspoon fresh thyme leaves
2 bay leaves
Sprinkling of freshly grated nutmeg
1 teaspoon ground allspice
Minced chilli in oil according to taste
1.5kg/3lb 5oz pumpkin with top and bottom sliced off, quartered, peeled, seeds removed, and the flesh coarsely chopped
1.5 litres/6 cups allergy-free vegetable stock (bouillon) or 2 teaspoons allergy-free vegetable bouillon powder dissolved in boiling water
Sea salt and freshly ground black pepper

Creole seeds
1 teaspoon paprika
½ teaspoon ground cumin
½ teaspoon mixed spice* (pie spice)
60g/⅓ cup pumpkin seeds
175g/1 cup canned or frozen, unsweetened, sweetcorn kernels, drained or defrosted

* coeliacs please use gluten-free ingredients

Gently cook the onion in 1 tablespoon of oil in a large pan over a low heat until soft, but do not let them brown. Add the garlic, cumin seeds, thyme, bay leaves, nutmeg, allspice and chilli and stir together for 1 minute. Stir in the pumpkin, cover with the vegetable stock (bouillon) and bring to the boil over a medium heat. Simmer the soup for about 40 minutes, or until the pumpkin is soft.

Prepare the Creole seeds. Mix the paprika, ground cumin, mixed spice (pie spice) and the remaining oil together in a little bowl and toss the seeds in the mixture. Fry them in a non-stick pan with the sweetcorn for about 3–4 minutes until dark brown at the edges.

Leave the soup to cool and then purée in a blender until smooth. Transfer the soup back to the pan, reheat and season to taste with pepper. Stir in the hot Creole seeds and sweetcorn and serve immediately.

Summer Cooler Soup

This soup is a triumph for those of us who prefer 'no-cooking' recipes for summer dinner parties. When you are feeding just a few people, halve the quantities, keep the leftover soup chilled, then fill a thermos with some and take it to lunch with you over the next day or two.

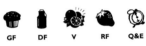

GF   DF   V   RF   Q&E

Serves 8

1 head crisp celery, carefully trimmed of leaves, root, blemishes and all tough fibres then coarsely chopped
1 litre/4 cups organic, pure tomato juice
1 large firm cucumber, peeled and coarsely chopped
700ml/2¾ cups organic, fresh or bottled carrot juice
1 small bunch spring onions (scallions), very finely chopped
1 large garlic clove, crushed
Chilli sauce* or minced chilli in vegetable oil
Juice of 1 lemon (or according to taste)
Sea salt and freshly ground black pepper
15g/½oz fresh parsley, finely chopped

* coeliacs please use gluten-free ingredients

Purée the prepared celery with the tomato juice in a blender, at the highest speed, until smooth. Pour it into a big serving bowl. Purée the cucumber with the carrot juice until smooth and add to the tomato and celery juice mixture in the bowl.

Sprinkle the soup with the spring onions (scallions), garlic, chilli and lemon juice and then stir and season to taste with salt and pepper.

Cover and chill until needed. Serve the soup chilled in soup bowls and sprinkle with the parsley.

The Big Book of Wheat-Free Cooking

Coconut and Tomato Soup

I made this by sheer accident one evening when I was rooting around the store cupboard, having run out of immediate ideas for dinner. As we love anything Thai or Indian, this seemed a rather good blend and has been made on many occasions since. The good news is that it can be served either hot or cold.

GF   DF   V   RF   Q&E

Serves 4

1 large onion, finely chopped

1 tablespoon cold pressed extra virgin olive oil

2 teaspoons ground cumin

1 teaspoon ground coriander

1 teaspoon mixed spice (pie spice)*

1 litre/4 cups organic, pure tomato juice

3 teaspoons allergy-free vegetable bouillon powder

400ml/14fl oz can reduced-fat coconut milk (Blue Dragon)

Sea salt and freshly ground black pepper

7g/¼oz fresh coriander (cilantro) leaves, chopped

Optional

A little minced chilli in oil or a chilli sauce*

* coeliacs please use gluten-free ingredients

Cook the onion in the oil with all the spices and chilli until softened, over a fairly low heat so that the onion does not brown. Increase the heat to medium, add the tomato juice and bouillon powder and stir occasionally while it is simmering. After about 20 minutes remove from the heat, stir in the coconut milk and leave to cool before puréeing in a blender until smooth.

Reheat the soup over a medium heat for about 10 minutes, seasoning with salt, pepper and more chilli if necessary. Serve with a sprinkling of fresh coriander (cilantro). Alternatively, transfer the soup to a bowl, cool, cover and chill until needed.

Pasta and Bean Soup

We often have this soup as a meal in itself. It is a healthy, warming winter lunch or Sunday-night supper for all the family. The Italians have all sorts of pastas that could be used for this dish, but it will be just as authentic if you use wheat-free macaroni, or you could break up some wheat-free tagliatelle. This soup can be frozen.

OPTIONAL

GF   DF   V   RF

Serves 4–6

---

2 x 400g/14oz cans borlotti beans or 455g/1lb dried ones, soaked for 12 hours

1 tablespoon cold pressed extra virgin olive oil and some extra for serving

85g/3oz chopped pancetta, or diced streaky, rindless smoked bacon (not for vegetarian or reduced fat option)

1 large carrot, peeled and diced

1 onion, diced

2 celery sticks, diced

2 slim leeks, sliced

2 small red chillies (strength according to taste), chopped

1 teaspoon chopped rosemary

14 sage leaves, shredded

2 bay leaves

750ml/3 cups or 1 bottle good-quality tomato pasta sauce

1 litre/4 cups cold water (use some to rinse out the tomato sauce bottle)

1 tablespoon allergy-free vegetable bouillon powder

2 large garlic cloves, crushed

150g/1¾ cups wheat-free pasta* (macaroni or small-sized pasta)

110g/1½ cups French beans, cut into thirds

110g/¾ cup frozen peas

Sea salt and freshly ground black pepper

15g/½oz fresh parsley, chopped

---

* coeliacs please use gluten-free ingredients

If using canned beans, rinse them thoroughly and drain. If using dried beans, rinse them in cold water then cook in unsalted boiling water for about 1½ hours until just soft.

Heat the oil in a large heavy pan, add the pancetta or the bacon if you are using it, and cook for a few minutes until it turns golden. Add the carrot, onion, celery, leeks, chillies and herbs. Alternatively, just heat the oil and add the vegetables, chillies and herbs.

Continue to cook for about 3 minutes until the vegetables colour, then add the tomato sauce, water, bouillon powder and garlic, and cook for another 5 minutes. Stir in the borlotti beans and simmer for 30 minutes. Halfway through the cooking time, bring a pan of water to the boil and cook the pasta until al dente, drain and add to the soup.

Meanwhile, cook the French beans and the peas together in boiling water until just cooked through, drain and add to the soup. Season to taste with salt and pepper, sprinkle with the parsley and serve piping hot with a swirl of olive oil.

If the soup doesn't have enough liquid just add some more water or stock (bouillon), as it is a very adaptable soup and can expand to suit a sudden influx of guests!

Gingered Chicken Soup

Singles or couples could halve the quantities and enjoy this soup over several days. As with all chicken and stock dishes, allow it to get cold and then keep it chilled in the refrigerator until you need it. You can reboil the soup and add fresh bean sprouts, so it is a very good stand-by. You can also freeze this into portions and use for a quick lunch or appetizer.

A boiling chicken is the best thing for chicken soup, but they are increasingly hard to find. An ordinary roasting bird will be fine, but you must remove the meat after an hour or it will be too dry.

GF   DF   RF

Serves 10

Stock (bouillon)
1 boiling chicken, or an ordinary medium-sized roasting chicken, about 1.5kg/3lbs
2 litres/8 cups water plus 1 litre/4 cups for topping up
Pinch of sea salt and 1 teaspoon black peppercorns
1 tablespoon cold pressed extra virgin olive oil
6cm/2in piece root ginger, peeled and cut into chunks
1 large onion, coarsely chopped
2 tablespoons Thai fish sauce*

Soup
6cm/2in piece root ginger, peeled and grated
Pinch of sea salt
1 garlic clove, crushed
1 small chilli (hot or mild according to taste), finely chopped
300g/5 cups bean sprouts
8 spring onions (scallions), finely chopped
15g/½oz fresh coriander (cilantro) leaves, finely chopped

Optional
Soy sauce* to serve

* coeliacs please use gluten-free ingredients

Put the chicken into a large pan and add the water, salt and peppercorns. Bring to the boil over a high heat. In a frying pan (skillet), heat 1 tablespoon of oil and stir in the ginger and onion until they begin to colour slightly, and then add them to the chicken. When the water is boiling, add 1 tablespoon of the Thai fish sauce, turn the heat down and leave the chicken to simmer. Remove the chicken after an hour and, when it is cool enough, pick off the meat and shred it coarsely. Put the carcass back into the pot and simmer for another 2 hours.

Strain the stock (bouillon) into a bowl and discard the carcass. When the stock (bouillon) is cold, cover and refrigerate it for at least 3 hours or overnight. You will then be able to skim off the layer of fat.

You can make this stock (bouillon) 1 day in advance; just make sure the shredded chicken meat is kept in an airtight container in the refrigerator or it will become dry. When you want to make the soup, bring the stock (bouillon) to the boil and let it simmer, adding the shredded chicken, another tablespoon of fish sauce, the grated ginger, salt, garlic and chilli. Stir in the bean sprouts and cook for 1 minute.

Serve the soup in warm bowls and top with the coriander (cilantro) and spring onions (scallions). As some people like to sprinkle their soup with soy sauce, serve it separately.

Beetroot and Cranberry Soup

Centuries ago, beetroot (beet) was grown for its leaves and not for the root. It was used to cure all sorts of ills. Most people throw away the leaves now, but they are a perfectly good substitute for spinach. This soup freezes well.

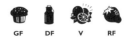

Serves 6

GF DF V RF

---

3 large fresh beetroots (beets), cooked in boiling water until tender, about 40 minutes, or 2 × 200g/7oz
   packets organic, cooked, whole beetroots (beets) (not in vinegar)
1 tablespoon cold pressed extra virgin olive oil
1 large onion, chopped
150g/5oz cranberries, fresh or frozen, or when out of season 40g/⅓ cup dried cranberries
Pinch of ground cloves
Pinch of grated nutmeg
Pinch of cayenne pepper
Freshly ground black pepper
2 teaspoons allergy-free vegetable bouillon powder
1 litre/4 cups cranberry juice (Ocean Spray or similar)
Finely grated rind and juice of ½ an unwaxed orange
6 teaspoons half-fat crème fraîche or dairy-free Sour Supreme (see page 305 for stockist) for serving
15g/½oz chopped coriander (cilantro) leaves for serving

If using fresh beetroots (beets), top and tail them and peel them once they have cooled down. Discard the skins, stalks and the cooking liquid. Quarter either the fresh or the prepared beetroots (beets). Cook the beetroots (beets) and onion with the oil in a pan over medium heat for about 5 minutes. Stir frequently to prevent the vegetables sticking to the pan.

Add the cranberries, spices, bouillon powder and cranberry juice, bring to the boil and then reduce the heat slightly and simmer it for about 30 minutes. When the onions are soft, remove the pan from the heat, add both the orange rind and juice and adjust the seasoning with the pepper.

Once the soup is cool, purée until smooth in a blender, return to the pan and reheat. Serve hot with a spoonful of crème fraîche or Sour Supreme and a sprinkling of coriander (cilantro) in each bowl.

Artichoke Chowder

This is a slight variation on a traditional chowder. The artichokes give the soup a very smooth and subtle flavour.

Serves 4

GF   DF   V   RF

Juice of ½ a lemon
500g/1lb 2oz Jerusalem artichokes, peeled and coarsely chopped
1 small onion, finely chopped
1 large baking potato, peeled and chopped into small cubes
1 leek, severely trimmed and finely chopped
1 tablespoon cold pressed extra virgin olive oil
1 teaspoon fresh thyme leaves
1 bay leaf
1 litre/4 cups hot allergy-free vegetable stock (bouillon)
A sprinkling of grated nutmeg
Sea salt and freshly ground black pepper
1 heaped tablespoon chopped fresh parsley leaves

Squeeze the lemon into a bowl of cold water and as you peel and chop the artichokes, submerge them in the water to prevent discolouration.

Gently cook the onions, potatoes and leeks together in the oil in a pan over a low heat. Do not let them brown and ensure that they are softened before adding the thyme, bay leaf and artichokes. Cover with the stock (bouillon) and simmer for 40 minutes or until the artichokes are soft. Let the soup cool and then purée in a blender until smooth. Transfer the soup back to the pan and cook for a further 5 minutes over a medium heat stirring all the time.

Season to taste with nutmeg and pepper, and remove from the heat. Serve sprinkled with the chopped parsley. This soup is very long-suffering and can be reheated again over several days, but sprinkle it with a little fresh parsley each time. (Always cool the soup, cover and chill in the refrigerator.)

Canapés, Appetizers and Snacks ...

Parmesan Biscuits with Smoked Salmon and Crème Fraîche

These biscuits are very quick to make and can be topped with anything you fancy – for a vegetarian alternative try crème fraîche with a tiny dollop of pesto and a strip of roasted pepper. The biscuits can also be frozen, which makes them ideal for Christmas entertaining.

GF

Makes 12 biscuits (double the ingredients for Christmas menu on page 295)

Parmesan biscuits
85g/¾ cup wheat-free flour mix*
1 heaped teaspoon wheat-free baking powder*
½ teaspoon fine salt
55g/1⅔ cup finely grated Parmesan cheese
1 large organic free-range egg
2 tablespoons cold pressed extra virgin olive oil
1 tablespoon organic milk
A little organic milk or beaten egg for brushing

Topping
12 heaped teaspoons half-fat crème fraîche
12 small pieces smoked salmon
12 little sprigs fresh dill
A little lemon juice
A little cayenne pepper
A scattering of rocket (arugula) and a little cold pressed extra virgin olive oil to serve

6cm/2½ in round fluted pastry cutter

*coeliacs please use gluten-free ingredients

The Big Book of Wheat-Free Cooking

Preheat the oven to 190°C/375°F/Gas mark 5.

Sift the flour into a food processor and add the other biscuit ingredients, except the milk. Mix until blended then add enough milk to make a soft dough. Turn the dough out onto a floured board and shape into a ball. At this stage you can wrap and either chill or freeze the dough for future use.

Roll the dough out to a thickness of about 1cm/½ in and cut into rounds with the cutter. Roll out the trimmings to make the next batch. Place the biscuits on a baking tray, brush them with a little milk or beaten egg and bake for about 10 minutes until golden. Cool for a few moments and transfer the biscuits to a wire rack to cool completely.

You can also freeze them at this stage and reheat before using.

Place two biscuits on each plate and spoon a dollop of crème fraîche on top of each. Cover with a generous slice of smoked salmon, twisted nicely to sit on top of the crème fraîche. Top it with a little sprig of dill, sprinkle with a little lemon juice and dust with a little cayenne pepper. Arrange a small handful of rocket (arugula) leaves around the biscuits and serve with a drizzle of oil.

Mini Potato Pancakes with Smoked Trout and Salsa

These pancakes can be frozen, which makes them an ideal Christmas appetizer – simply warm them through, top them and serve. You can change the topping to rare roast beef topped with a dollop of crème fraîche, mixed with horseradish and black pepper. Alternatively, how about using smoked mackerel in the same way and serve it with chopped dill? For a vegetarian option, simply swap the smoked trout for slices of roast sweet peppers (bell peppers). The pancakes are also delicious spread simply with butter or dairy-free margarine.

Makes 18–20 canapés or serves 6 as an appetizer
(double the ingredients for New Year's Eve menu on page 295)

GF   DF   RF   Q&E

Pancakes
340g/12oz floury potatoes, such as King Edward, peeled and cut into large chunks
Sea salt
115g/1 heaped cup wheat-free flour mix*
Cold pressed extra virgin olive oil for cooking

Topping
18–20 heaped teaspoons half-fat crème fraîche or Tofutti dairy-free Creamy Smooth cream-style cheese (see page 305 for stockist)
2 large fillets of skinless smoked trout
170g/6oz tub fresh salsa* (can be frozen until needed)

Optional
Some rocket (arugula) and extra virgin olive oil

5cm/2in round metal pastry cutter

* coeliacs please use gluten-free ingredients

Bring a pan of water to the boil, add the potatoes and cook until soft. Drain the potatoes in a colander set over the pan, cover with a tea towel and leave to steam dry for 5 minutes. Mash the potatoes in a bowl with a pinch of salt until smooth.

Gradually beat the flour into the potatoes using a wooden spoon; you may have to use your hands towards the end, as the dough may be very thick. Knead the dough lightly on a floured board. Cut in half and roll out to a thickness of 5mm/¼in. Use your cutter to stamp out 5cm/2in rounds. Knead the dough remnants gently back into the remaining ball of dough, roll out again and repeat until all the dough is used up.

Brush a large non-stick frying pan (skillet) with some oil, place it over a medium heat and cook the pancakes on one side until they are firm enough to flip over and are tinged with golden brown. You will need to cook them in batches. Cool the pancakes on a wire rack lined with non-stick baking parchment (wax paper).

You can layer the pancakes in non-stick baking parchment (wax paper), wrap them in kitchen foil and freeze until needed. Defrost and bake for about 3–5 minutes in a hot oven.

Decorate the serving plates with some rocket (arugula) and a drizzle of oil. Arrange three pancakes on each plate and top each with a dollop of the crème fraîche or dairy-free sour cream. Decorate with a generous piece of smoked trout and sprinkle with a pinch of pepper. If you are serving them as an appetizer, spoon a neat pile of salsa on the edge of one of the pancakes and serve immediately. To serve them as canapés, top each pancake with a blob of salsa.

Smoked Salmon and Crab Timbales

This is a very easy and useful appetizer for special parties because you can make it in the morning and simply turn the timbales out onto plates a few minutes before sitting down to eat. Walnut Bread* and Rye and Barley Soda Bread* (see pages 273 and 271) are both delicious with the salmon.

Makes 4–5   GF   DF   RF   Q&E

170g/6oz packet smoked salmon

170g/6oz fresh, canned or frozen and defrosted white crab meat

2 heaped tablespoons reduced-fat mayonnaise* (check the label for added wheat)

4 teaspoons lemon juice

Sea salt and freshly ground black pepper

4 ripe vine tomatoes, peeled

15g/½oz fresh dill, finely chopped

1 small ripe avocado

1 teaspoon red wine vinegar

3 tablespoons cold pressed extra virgin olive oil

A pinch of unrefined golden caster (superfine) sugar

A couple of handfuls of rocket leaves (arugula) for decoration

5 standard-sized ramekins or individual metal pudding basins lined with clingfilm (plastic wrap)

* coeliacs please use gluten-free ingredients

Lay the smoked salmon on a board and using a round pastry cutter the same size as the ramekins, cut out two rounds for each one. Place one round of salmon at the bottom of each lined ramekin. Keep the remaining rounds to one side and chop up all the remaining salmon.

Drain the crab meat if it is canned. Place the crab meat in a small bowl and stir in the mayonnaise, salmon bits, 2 teaspoons of the lemon juice and the seasoning. Put a spoonful into each ramekin – this should use up only half the mixture.

Quarter the tomatoes and remove the seeds. Place the seeds in a small sieve over a bowl and leave to one side. Chop the tomatoes, season, add a little chopped dill and divide between the ramekins. Peel and chop the avocado, sprinkle it with the remaining lemon juice and a little seasoning and spoon over the tomatoes. Divide the remaining crab between the ramekins and top with the remaining salmon rounds. Cover tightly with clingfilm (plastic wrap) and chill the timbales for 2–12 hours.

Over a bowl, gently stir the tomato seeds and pulp in the sieve so that you have a few spoonfuls of juice. Discard the seeds. Stir the vinegar, oil, a little salt, pepper and a pinch of sugar in to the juice to make a dressing.

To serve the timbales, turn each one onto a plate, drizzle the dressing around it and decorate with a few rocket (arugula) leaves. Serve with wheat- or gluten-free bread and butter or dairy-free margarine.

Spicy Prawn Poppadums

This has to be the quickest canapé recipe ever – it takes just a few minutes. The quantity this recipe makes is fine for about 16 guests, so double, treble or quadruple the quantities as required. For a vegetarian alternative, use folded strips of roasted pepper (bell pepper) instead of the prawns (shrimp).

Makes 55

GF   DF

---

55 cooked and peeled large prawns (shrimp), thawed and drained if frozen

55 ready-to-eat mini poppadums, in any flavour or, if they are unavailable, use Orgran or Blue Dragon rice crackers (check the labels to ensure the product is gluten-free)

250ml/1 cup half-fat crème fraîche or Tofutti dairy-free Sour Supreme (see page 305 for stockist)

55 fresh coriander (cilantro) leaves

Optional

Some fresh rocket (arugula) to decorate the serving plate

Rinse and dry the prawns (shrimp) and keep covered in the refrigerator until needed. Within 2 hours of your party, lay out the poppadums or rice crackers on a serving tray that you can decorate with the rocket (arugula). At the last minute, spoon a small dollop of crème fraîche or Sour Supreme onto each poppadum. Place a prawn (shrimp) at a jaunty angle on each poppadum and decorate with a coriander (cilantro) leaf.

Cannellini Bean and Tomato Crostini

This is a very superior beans on toast! White bread is definitely the best choice for the toast as it absorbs the oil well and its less distinctive taste allows the taste of the topping to dominate.

GF **DF** **Q&E**

Serves 2

1 small red onion, very finely chopped

1 tablespoon cold pressed extra virgin olive oil and extra for drizzling

1 garlic clove, crushed

130g/4½oz pack cubetti di pancetta or finely chopped rindless bacon

300g/10½oz can cannellini beans, drained and rinsed

1 large vine tomato, cored and coarsely chopped

1 heaped teaspoon chopped rosemary or sage leaves

Sea salt and freshly ground black pepper

2 heaped tablespoons chopped fresh parsley

2 very thick slices of crustless white wheat- and gluten-free bread (see page 304 for stockist)

Some freshly grated Parmesan or dairy-free Florentino Parmazano (see page 306 for stockist) to serve

Heat the oil in a frying pan (skillet), add the onion and fry over low heat until it is soft. Stir in the garlic and pancetta or bacon and cook for about 5 minutes until the onions are golden and the pancetta or bacon is crispy. Add the beans, tomato, rosemary or sage and season to taste. Heat through for about 5 minutes then sprinkle with parsley.

Meanwhile, toast the slices of bread and place on warm plates. Spoon the bean mixture over the top, drizzle with extra oil and sprinkle with some Parmesan or Parmazano.

Welsh Rarebit

I have to admit the idea of doing a wheat-free version of this recipe comes solely from my husband, who asked if we could have it for lunch one day as he had enjoyed it with a pint of Guinness in a local pub. I find it amazing that such an easy recipe has not, until now, been included in any of my cookbooks. It is also delicious cut into fingers and served in a bowl of French onion soup – a truly European combination!

Serves 2

GF   **V**   **Q&E**

30g/1oz organic butter

½ small red onion, finely chopped

115g/4oz piece extra strong organic Cheddar cheese, grated

80ml/⅓ cup ale (coeliacs can use very dry cider)

A pinch of sea salt and freshly ground black pepper

1 teaspoon mustard*

2 organic free-range eggs, lightly beaten

4 thick slices wheat-free white bread (see page 304 for stockist)

* coeliacs please use gluten-free ingredients

Melt the butter in a heavy-based saucepan, stir in the onion and cook gently, over low heat, until soft. Stir in the cheese, ale, seasoning and mustard and cook gently until combined and melted. Stir in the beaten eggs and let the mixture thicken slightly – this will take about 2–3 minutes but don't overcook it or you will end up with scrambled eggs!

    Toast the bread on both sides, spoon the cheese mixture over each slice and grill (broil) until golden and puffed. Serve immediately.

Stuffed Mushrooms

These mushrooms can be served as an appetizer, a snack or as a main course for two. They also cook brilliantly on a barbecue.

Serves 4

4 large, open-cap field mushrooms, stalks removed and discarded
Cold pressed extra virgin olive oil for brushing
Sea salt and freshly ground black pepper
4 teaspoons truffle oil
4 thin red onion slices, the same size as the mushrooms
1 mozzarella, about 155g/5½oz, cut into 4 slices
A handful of basil leaves, finely sliced
4 large tomato slices, the same size as the mushrooms
2 heaped tablespoons wheat-free breadcrumbs*

Optional
Baby rocket (arugula) and/or spinach leaves tossed with a little olive oil and black pepper to serve

* coeliacs please use gluten-free ingredients

Preheat the oven to 200°C/400°F/Gas mark 6.

Brush the caps with olive oil and place them gill-side up on a baking tray. Season and drizzle with truffle oil. Place a slice of onion inside the cavity of each mushroom and then a layer of mozzarella, some basil, a slice of tomato, some breadcrumbs, more basil and a drizzle of olive oil.

Cook in the oven for about 15 minutes until the mushrooms are softened and the cheese has melted. Serve immediately on a bed of rocket (arugula) or baby spinach leaves.

Tomato and Pesto Tarts

These very cute little tarts are ideal for picnics and lunches al fresco. They can also be served as a perfect appetizer at parties. Ensure you use vine tomatoes because their taste is so superior and this always matters in simple recipes.

GF   V

Serves 8–9

Pastry
200g/1¾ cups wheat-free flour mix*
125g/4½oz organic butter or dairy-free margarine, cut into 8 pieces
Pinch of sea salt
1 organic free-range egg
A little cold water

Filling
9 medium-sized, vine-ripe tomatoes, stalks removed, and each one scratched with a sharp knife and immersed in a bowl of boiling water for 5 minutes or until the skins peel off with ease
120g/4oz tub fresh deli-made pesto or a bottled organic pesto
Freshly ground black pepper
About 60g/2oz pecorino cheese shavings (or other sheep's cheese)
Pinch of cayenne pepper

Optional
Basil leaves to decorate

3 x 6-cup mini tart trays

* *coeliacs please use gluten-free ingredients*

The Big Book of Wheat-Free Cooking

Preheat the oven to 180°C/350°F/Gas mark 4.

Make the pastry in a food processor. Put all the pastry ingredients, except the water, in the processor and whizz for a few seconds until the mixture resembles breadcrumbs. Gradually add the water, processing briefly until the mixture comes together into a ball of dough.

Remove the dough, wrap it in clingfilm (plastic wrap) and freeze for 10 minutes. Meanwhile peel off the tomato skins, cut the tops off and discard.

Roll out the dough into a medium–thick pastry on a floured board and then cut into 18 circles. Line the cups of the baking tray with the pastry circles and prick the bases with a fork.

Quarter each tomato, removing the white core and attached seeds, which you can discard. Place a double thickness of absorbent kitchen paper on a clean surface and lay the tomatoes on top. Cover with another double layer, which will soak up the excess juices. Slice the tomatoes into smaller pieces that you can arrange nicely in each pastry case. Divide the tomatoes between the pastry cases and season them with a little black pepper. Spoon about a teaspoon of the pesto over the top of each tomato-filled tart, then sprinkle with pecorino shavings and cayenne pepper. Bake them in the oven for about 25 minutes until the pastry is golden and the filling is bubbling.

Let the tarts cool down and when they are just cool enough to handle, lift them out of the tray. Serve the tarts straightaway, two on each plate, decorated with some basil leaves.

Vegetable Spring Rolls

These spring rolls are uncooked and therefore easy to make, as well as being healthy. You can either serve them as an appetizer, or as a main course with a bowl of steamed fragrant Thai rice. The rice wrappers are available from large supermarkets or Chinese grocery stores.

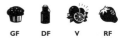

Serves 4

GF   DF   V   RF

Spring rolls

1 small red pepper (bell pepper), seeded and cut into very fine julienne strips

Drizzle of cold pressed extra virgin olive oil

110g/4oz bean sprouts, blanched for 1 minute in boiling water, drained and refreshed under cold running water

¼ small cucumber, peeled, seeded and cut into fine julienne strips

1 medium carrot, peeled and cut into fine julienne strips

2 spring onions (scallions), cut into very fine strips

7g/¼oz each mint, coriander (cilantro) and basil leaves, coarsely chopped

60g/⅓ cup roasted, salted almonds, crushed

Freshly ground black pepper

2 packets rice wrappers (12)

Dipping sauce

Juice of 2 limes

2 tablespoons soy sauce*

4 teaspoons rice or sherry vinegar

Minced chilli in oil or dried flaked chillies

2 tablespoons clear runny honey

3 teaspoons sesame seeds

4 tablespoons tomato ketchup

* coeliacs please use gluten-free ingredients

First make the rolls. Stir-fry the peppers in the oil in a pan for a few minutes and leave to cool. Mix the peppers with the bean sprouts, cucumber, carrot, spring onions (scallions), herbs and nuts in a bowl. Season with pepper but not salt, as you are already using salted almonds.

Dip a rice wrapper in warm water until it is pliable and then place on a very wet tea towel on a clean surface. Generously pile a line of the vegetable mixture along the lower edge. Roll the rice wrapper away from you, tucking in the ends as you go. If you dip your fingers in water this prevents the rolls from getting sticky. Place each roll seam-side down on a serving plate. Make up each roll in the same way.

To make the dipping sauce, mix the ingredients together in a small saucepan, bring to the boil and boil the sauce for about 30 seconds. Drizzle it all over the plate of spring rolls or serve alongside. You can decorate this dish with some exotic flower heads or leaves and serve immediately.

Wrapped Asparagus with Quick Hollandaise Sauce

This classic appetizer also makes a super quick lunch dish if you follow the asparagus with a fresh mixed salad with herbs, warm wheat-free bread and a selection of goats' cheeses.

GF   DF   Q&E

Serves 4

Asparagus
455g/1lb fresh asparagus, trimmed
4 slices Serrano ham
Cold pressed extra virgin olive oil
Freshly ground black pepper

Quick hollandaise sauce
115g/4oz organic butter or dairy-free margarine
2 large organic free-range egg yolks
1 tablespoon white wine vinegar
1 teaspoon fresh lemon juice
A pinch of unrefined golden caster (superfine) sugar
A pinch of sea salt

Blanch the asparagus in boiling water for 3 minutes, drain and plunge into a bowl of cold filtered water.

Put the butter or margarine into a small pan and melt until boiling over medium heat. Meanwhile, blend the egg yolks with the vinegar, lemon juice, sugar and sea salt in a food processor. Pour the boiling fat into the eggs, blending all the time until the sauce is thick. Transfer the hollandaise sauce to a little serving bowl and place in the centre of a large plate.

Drain the asparagus, divide the spears into 4 portions and wrap each portion in a slice of ham.

Place on a baking tray, brush with oil and grill (broil) until the ham is crispy. Season with a little pepper and serve around the bowl of hollandaise sauce.

Broad Beans on Lemon Crostini

You may think it is such a bore to peel the beans but it really is worth it, not only are they sweet and tender but they are a lovely, cheerful bright green. This dish is ideal for lunch al fresco, or as an appetizer.

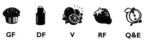

Serves 2

GF   DF   V   RF   Q&E

255g/9oz frozen or fresh baby broad (fava) beans

2 garlic cloves, crushed

Sea salt and freshly ground black pepper

2 tablespoons cold pressed extra virgin olive oil, plus plenty extra for sprinkling

7g/¼oz coarsely chopped flat-leaf parsley

15g/½oz fresh basil leaves, shredded

2 white wheat-free bread rolls*, refreshed according to instructions on the packet, tops sliced off and discarded or 1 small wheat-free baguette*, refreshed according to the instructions on the packet, and then halved horizontally (see page 304 for stockist)

Juice of ½ a lemon

* coeliacs please use gluten-free ingredients

Cook the broad (fava) beans in boiling water for about 3 minutes and drain. Once they are cool enough to handle, pop them from their skins. Discard the skins and put the beans into a small pan.

Add the garlic, salt and pepper and the 2 tablespoons of olive oil. Gently stew the beans for about 5 minutes, add the herbs and cook for another 3 minutes.

Place the prepared bread on to two plates and spoon the beans and oil over each one. Squeeze over the lemon juice, drizzle with plenty of extra virgin olive oil, so that the bread absorbs it, and then sprinkle with pepper and serve.

Sweet Red Pepper Dip

Suitably pink for St Valentine's Day, this dip can be as extravagant or as simple as you like. For the best effect, serve the dip in a glass bowl in the middle of a large glass dish, surrounded by your chosen dippers. You can dip cooked king prawns (jumbo shrimp) or voluptuous barely cooked scallops, lightly cooked asparagus tips or grilled baby courgettes (zucchini). The leftover dip is delicious for lunch the next day.

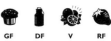

Serves 4

3 red peppers (bell peppers), seeded and coarsely chopped
1 red onion, coarsely chopped
1 teaspoon fresh thyme leaves
1 garlic clove, crushed
1 tablespoon cold pressed extra virgin olive oil
1 tablespoon balsamic vinegar
Sea salt and freshly ground black pepper
1 finely chopped chilli (choose your own preferred strength)
125ml/½ cup 50% reduced-fat crème fraîche, chilled or dairy-free natural (plain) set yogurt

To serve
455g/1lb fresh asparagus, lightly cooked in boiling water until al dente, drained, refreshed under cold running water
Or, less expensively, 1 packet organic yellow 100% corn chips

Cook the peppers and onions in a saucepan over a medium heat with the thyme, garlic and oil for about 10 minutes, stirring occasionally. Add the balsamic vinegar, salt, pepper and chilli and continue to cook for another 15 minutes until they are browned, soft and mushy.

Leave the mixture to cool and then purée in a blender. Transfer the mixture to a bowl and when it is cold, stir in the crème fraîche or yogurt and adjust the seasoning to taste.

Spoon the dip into a bowl, cover and chill until needed. Serve it with the asparagus or corn chips.

Fish and Seafood ...

Roast Skate with Baby Summer Vegetables

Skate is so easy to cook and looks more interesting than a slab of fish. Here it is lightly cooked with tiny vegetables for a healthy and light summer dish. In winter, I use whatever frozen baby vegetables I can find.

GF   DF   Q&E

Serves 4

24 tiny new potatoes

170g/6oz miniature, trimmed baby leeks or baby carrots, topped and tailed

155g/5½oz trimmed asparagus spears or fine green beans, topped and tailed

170g/6oz mangetout or sugar snap peas or halved baby courgettes (zucchini)

4 tablespoons wheat-free flour mix*

Sea salt and freshly ground black pepper

4 medium-sized skate wings

2 tablespoons cold pressed extra virgin olive oil

115g/4oz organic butter or dairy-free margarine

16 whole fresh sage leaves

4 tablespoons chopped fresh flat-leaf parsley

Juice of 1 large lemon

1 unwaxed lemon, cut into quarters for decoration

*coeliacs please use gluten-free ingredients

Preheat the oven to 200°C/400°F/Gas mark 6.

Bring a pan of water to the boil, add the potatoes and cook until nearly soft before adding the other vegetables. Add the remaining vegetables in stages so that the leeks or carrots are nearly cooked through before adding the green beans or courgettes (zucchini). The asparagus and mangetout or sugar snaps should be the last to cook, as all the vegetables must remain crunchy. Drain the vegetables and keep to one side.

Season the flour with salt and pepper and spread over a plate. Coat the skate wings with the mixture and shake off the excess. Add the oil and half the butter or margarine to a frying pan (skillet), add the fish and fry for 2 minutes on each side. Transfer the skate wings to a baking tray and bake for 15 minutes until crisp.

Halfway through the oven cooking time, add the remaining butter or margarine to the fish pan and, when it is foaming, stir in the sage and vegetables. Sauté them for 7 minutes, stirring occasionally. Stir in the parsley, season to taste with salt and pepper and sprinkle with lemon juice.

Remove the skate from the baking tray and set each piece on a warm plate. Spoon the summer vegetables around the fish and serve with a lemon quarter.

Trout in Oatmeal

We have a trout farm near us in Hampshire, which means I can buy freshly-caught fish and serve it with delicious, locally-grown watercress.

Serves 2

DF   Q&E

70g/½ cup medium or fine organic oatmeal
Sea salt, freshly ground black pepper and a sprinkling of cayenne pepper
2 thick, tail end, loch trout fillets (size according to appetites)
2 tablespoons cold pressed extra virgin olive oil
4 thick slices rindless, dry-cure back bacon
30g/1oz organic butter or dairy-free margarine
1 unwaxed lemon, cut into 4 wedges

Spoon the oatmeal onto a plate and season with salt, pepper and cayenne. Coat the trout in the oatmeal and gently shake off the excess.

Warm half the oil in a large non-stick frying pan (skillet), add the bacon and cook until tinged with gold. Move the bacon to the side of the pan, add the remaining oil and the trout fillets and cook over medium heat until they are dark gold. Now add the butter or margarine and cook the other side until crispy and light brown. Drain the trout and the bacon on absorbent kitchen paper and serve with wedges of lemon and fresh, wheat-free bread and butter or dairy-free margarine.

The Big Book of Wheat-Free Cooking

Super Cheat's Fish Pie

This is the quickest fish pie I have ever made therefore it's made frequently! You can change the fish to suit the season and budget, and you can use mussels or squid if you don't like asparagus and artichokes. If you prefer other crisps (chips), please check that they are not coated in either wheat or gluten.

Serves 4–6

GF   Q&E

225g/8oz skinned, boneless cod fillet (or any similar white fish)

225g/8oz skinned, boneless smoked haddock fillet

255g/9oz packet fresh large prawns (shrimp)

400g/14oz can artichoke hearts, drained

Sea salt and freshly ground black pepper

250ml/1 cup half-fat crème fraîche

2 tablespoons chopped fresh dill

170g/6oz fresh asparagus spears

155g/5½oz packet black pepper Kettle chips (or other gluten-free variety)

55g/2oz finely grated organic hard cheese (anything from Parmesan to Cheddar)

Cut the fresh and the smoked fish into generous bite-size pieces (don't make them too small or they'll disintegrate) and place in a large non-stick pan. Add the prawns (shrimp) and artichoke hearts and season lightly with salt and pepper. Stir in the crème fraîche and dill, place the pan over a low heat and shake the pan gently from time to time so that the fish and vegetables cook gently through – this takes about 15 minutes.

Meanwhile, cook the asparagus spears in boiling water until just soft, drain and then add to the fish mixture.

Adjust the seasoning as necessary and transfer the mixture to a hot ovenproof serving dish and smooth over. Sprinkle the fish mixture with the crisps (chips) and cheese. Grill (broil) the fish pie until the cheese is melted and golden then serve immediately.

Rosemary, Monkfish and Pancetta Kebabs

This is a very light, easy and summery dish so a simple salad and some new potatoes are the perfect accompaniments. You can use salmon, swordfish or tuna for a change, as long as the fish is thick enough to prevent it from dropping off the skewer during cooking.

Serves 2   GF   DF   Q&E

2 very thick slices white wheat-free bread*, crusts removed (see page 304 for stockist)
4 tablespoons cold pressed extra virgin olive oil
1 teaspoon finely chopped fresh rosemary
2 unwaxed lemons, the rind of one finely grated
Sea salt and freshly ground black pepper
340g/12oz trimmed monkfish tails, cut into 12 bite-size chunks
4 slices pancetta (prosciutto or Parma ham), cut into 2 long strips
Extra cold pressed extra virgin olive oil if necessary

2 long or 4 short wood or metal skewers (soak the wooden skewers in cold water for 10 minutes before using)

* coeliacs please use gluten-free ingredients

Cut the bread into generous bite-size pieces so that they will look good with the fish chunks.

In a small bowl, mix the oil, rosemary, lemon rind, salt and pepper together.

Wrap each chunk of fish in a strip of pancetta.

Thread the bread alternately with the monkfish onto the skewers until you have used up all the ingredients and have two or four full kebabs. Lightly brush the fish and bread with the oil mixture and set under a hot grill (broiler) or over the embers of a hot barbecue to cook. Turn the kebabs over four times so that each time a different edge of bread is toasted. Drizzle with extra olive oil if the kebabs become too dry. By the time the bread is golden and crispy on all sides the fish will be cooked through and ready to eat.

Quarter the remaining lemon and squeeze the juice over the fish as you eat it. Serve the kebabs with a big mixed salad and new potatoes or a rice salad.

Thai Seafood Casserole

You can freeze this dish. Let it defrost and then reheat gently so that the fish does not become over-cooked. Add the coriander (cilantro) to the casserole at the last moment.

GF **DF** **Q&E**

Serves 4

2 tablespoons cold pressed extra virgin olive oil
1 large onion, very finely chopped
1 long red chilli, seeded and finely sliced
2 garlic cloves, finely chopped
2.5cm/1in piece fresh root ginger, finely chopped
225g/8oz fine green beans, topped, tailed and halved
450ml/1¾ cups allergy-free fish stock (bouillon) or filtered water
2 heaped teaspoons red Thai Curry paste* (more or less according to preference)
A good pinch of dried kaffir lime leaves
4 ripe vine tomatoes, peeled, seeded and cut into thick slices
200ml/¾ cup coconut cream
590g/1lb 5oz bag frozen raw crayfish tails
A large handful of fresh coriander (cilantro) leaves, coarsely chopped

* coeliacs please use gluten-free ingredients

Heat the oil in a non-stick wok or very large frying pan (skillet), add the onions and cook them over medium heat until soft and golden. Stir in the chilli, garlic, ginger and green beans and cook for about a minute. Stir in the stock (bouillon), Thai curry paste and lime leaves, bring to the boil and simmer for about 3 minutes. Reduce the heat slightly, add the tomatoes and simmer for 5 minutes. Stir in the coconut cream, add the crayfish and cook for about 5 minutes until all the seafood is opaque. Stir in the coriander (cilantro) and serve with some rice – fragrant Thai rice is particularly good.

Salmon and Watercress en Croûte

Salmon en Croûte can be served warm or cold. It is delicious cold for a buffet – decorate the dish with rocket (arugula) or lambs lettuce (mâche) and serve accompanied by the sauce. You can double up on all the ingredients and make one large salmon and watercress en croûte for 12. For special occasions, serve with the Quick Hollandaise Sauce recipe on page 54 (you will need to double the given quantities to serve 6), baby new potatoes, asparagus, and a watercress, orange and toasted pine nut salad.

Serves 6

GF   DF

Pastry

155g/1½ cups organic rice flour
155g/1½ cups Orgran self-raising gluten-free flour (see page 305 for stockist)
155g/5½oz organic butter or dairy-free margarine
1 large organic free-range egg
A pinch of fine salt
Cold filtered water

Filling

710g/1lb 9oz fresh salmon, as two matching fillets, skinned and all bones removed
Sea salt and freshly ground black pepper
2 x 55g/2oz packets prepared watercress or a large bunch of watercress, trimmed (the watercress must be dry or you will have a runny filling)
155g/5½oz reduced-fat cream cheese (Philadelphia) or 225g/8oz Tofutti Creamy Smooth dairy-free alternative (see page 305 for stockist)
Finely grated rind of 1 unwaxed lemon
1 small organic free-range egg, beaten – to glaze the pastry

Sauce

500g/1lb 2oz half-fat crème fraîche or dairy-free Tofutti Sour Supreme (see page 305 for stockist)
2 tablespoons each finely chopped fresh parsley and chives
Sea salt and freshly ground black pepper
A little finely grated lemon rind with a good squeeze of lemon juice (according to taste) from an unwaxed lemon

Make the pastry first. In a food processor, briefly mix both the flours with the butter or margarine until it resembles breadcrumbs. Add the egg and salt and process briefly. Add a little water until the mixture comes into a ball of dough – the amount of water needed will depend on the absorbency of the flour you use. Remove the dough and place it on a floured board.

Meanwhile, sprinkle the salmon fillets with salt and pepper and set aside.

Make the filling in a food processor: finely chop the watercress and then add the dairy or dairy-free cream cheese, finely grated lemon and some salt and pepper and purée until smooth.

Cut the pastry dough in half and roll one half out on a floured board into a thin rectangle large enough to fit the fillet of salmon, with about 2.5cm/1in to spare around the edges – it should be approximately 35.5cm/13in long × 18cm/7in wide.

Place the rolled dough on a non-stick baking tray and lay one salmon fillet, skinned side down, in the centre of the pastry. Spread the filling over the salmon and cover with the remaining salmon fillet, skinned side up. Brush the pastry edges with beaten egg and cover the fish with the remaining rolled pastry. Pinch the edges together to seal and brush the pastry with the remaining beaten egg.

Gently score a crisscross pattern with a knife all over the pastry, cover and chill for 35 minutes (you can chill it all day if you wish to but not overnight).

Preheat the oven to 200°C/400°F/Gas mark 6.

Bake the salmon for 35–40 minutes until the pastry is golden brown and the fish is lightly cooked. Remove the salmon from the oven and leave to settle for 5 minutes. Mix the sauce ingredients together in a bowl and serve with the salmon or serve it with Quick Hollandaise Sauce (see page 54).

Crispy Squid in Breadcrumbs

You can freeze these squid rings so that you have them on hand for a quick dinner. I serve them with a healthy mixed salad and a tub of my favourite fresh salsa, which I also store in the deep-freeze.

GF   DF   Q&E

Serves 2

2 heaped tablespoons wheat-free flour mix* seasoned with sea salt, freshly ground black pepper and cayenne

1 large organic free-range egg, beaten

115g/1 heaped cup fine homemade wheat-free breadcrumbs* or Orgran gluten-free All Purpose Crumbs (see page 305 for stockist)

2 large squid, cleaned and cut into rings (use the tentacles if liked)

Enough sunflower oil to shallow fry

1 unwaxed lemon, quartered to serve

170g/6oz tub fresh salsa or either homemade garlic mayonnaise or tartare sauce

* coeliacs please use gluten-free alternatives

Place four plates in front of you. Put the seasoned flour on one, the beaten egg on the second, the crumbs on the third and keep the fourth plate empty.

Dip the prepared squid into the seasoned flour, then into the beaten egg and finally into the crumbs and pile them onto the fourth plate. Repeat until all the squid rings are coated.

Heat the oil in a large frying pan (skillet) and shallow fry about half the rings in one batch. Drain them on kitchen paper and keep them hot in the oven or on a hot plate whilst you quickly fry the remaining squid. Drain this last batch on kitchen paper. Serve the squid immediately with the lemon quarters and salsa.

Farfalle with Saffron, Prawns and Garlic

This pasta dish is a special treat as large prawns (shrimp) are expensive here in England. You can of course use a greater quantity of small prawns (shrimp), which would be cheaper and still delicious. A salad made up of baby spinach leaves, rocket (arugula), lambs lettuce (mâche) and fresh coriander (cilantro) makes an excellent sharp contrast to the rich sauce.

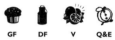

Serves 4   GF   DF   V   Q&E

250ml/1 cup single cream or Provamel dairy-free Soya Dream

A good pinch of saffron strands

1 garlic clove, finely chopped

225g/8oz tub or packet of cream cheese with garlic and herbs or dairy-free Tofutti creamy smooth cream cheese with garlic and herbs or French onion (see page 305 for stockist)

340g/12oz Orgran gluten-free farfalle (pasta bows) (see page 305 for stockist)

455g/1lb cooked peeled large prawns (shrimp)

2 tablespoons finely chopped fresh parsley

Sea salt and freshly ground black pepper

Bring a pan of salted water to the boil. Meanwhile, heat the cream, saffron, garlic and cream cheese together in a pan, over low heat, stirring constantly. As soon as it is smooth, let the sauce come to the boil and then remove it from the heat to infuse.

Cook the pasta until softened, stirring and separating the pasta from time to time. Drain the pasta and refresh with cold water. Refill the pan with salted water, bring it to the boil and cook the pasta until soft, stirring from time to time. (This method prevents the pasta becoming sticky.)

Meanwhile, gently reheat the cream mixture over low heat. Keep stirring the sauce so that it does not stick to the pan. Add the prawns (shrimp) and parsley and season to taste with salt and pepper.

Drain the pasta, toss in a warm serving bowl with the sauce and serve.

Tortelli with Tuna, Lemon and Caper Sauce

This is my emergency pasta dish, as I always have canned tuna and capers in my store cupboard and at least half a lemon lurking in the refrigerator somewhere.

A sprinkling of fresh parsley is lovely if you have some but otherwise simplicity is the best option. I serve the pasta with an olive, fennel and tomato salad.

Serves 2

GF   DF   V   Q&E

170g/6oz Orgran gluten-free tortelli (pasta shapes) (see page 305 for stockist)
Sea salt and freshly ground black pepper
200g/7oz can tuna fish in brine, drained and separated with a fork
Finely grated rind of 1 unwaxed lemon
1 tablespoon lemon juice
½ garlic clove, crushed and mixed with 3 tablespoons extra virgin olive oil
1 heaped tablespoon capers in wine vinegar*, drained and rinsed
A dash of chilli sauce* or chopped chilli in oil

Optional
Fresh flat-leaf parsley, coarsely chopped

* coeliacs please use gluten-free ingredients

Bring a pan of salted water to the boil. Add the tortelli and cook until softened, stirring and separating the pasta from time to time. Drain the pasta and refresh with cold water. Refill the pan with salted water, bring it to the boil and cook the pasta until soft, stirring from time to time. (This method prevents the pasta becoming sticky.)

Drain the pasta, toss in a warm serving bowl with the remaining ingredients and serve with the chopped parsley.

Fettuccini with Dill Cream and Avruga

I have heard that this pasta dish is sublime with real caviar but as this is rather out of my budget, I opt instead for Avruga, which is a good mock caviar. Serve the pasta with a continental salad.

GF · RF · Q&E

Serves 2

170g/6oz Orgran gluten-free fettuccini (see page 305 for stockist)
Sea salt and freshly ground black pepper
3 heaped tablespoons reduced-fat crème fraîche
7g/¼oz fresh dill, finely chopped
55g/2oz jar Avruga pasteurised herring roe (mock caviar)

Bring a pan of salted water to the boil, add the fettuccini and cook until softened, stirring and separating the pasta from time to time. Drain the pasta and refresh with cold water. Refill the pan with salted water, bring it to the boil and cook the pasta until soft, stirring from time to time. (This method prevents the pasta becoming sticky.)

Meanwhile, heat the crème fraîche and dill together in a medium-sized pan over very low heat, stirring constantly, until warmed through. Season to taste with salt and pepper.

Drain the pasta, toss in the pan of crème fraîche and spoon onto two warm plates. Serve with a dollop of mock – or real – caviar on top.

Roast Halibut with Rosemary and Breadcrumbs

This is a very quick and easy fish dish that you could also make with other firm white fish steaks. I keep breadcrumbs in bags in the deep-freeze so that the recipe is even quicker. If you have time, you can serve this dish with roasted vegetables such as courgettes (zucchini), sweet peppers (bell peppers) and aubergines (eggplant).

Serves 2

GF   DF   Q&E

2 large halibut steaks, rinsed clean under cold running water

1 teaspoon fresh or dried chopped rosemary

2 tablespoons cold pressed extra virgin olive oil

1 garlic clove, crushed

30g/1oz wheat-free breadcrumbs*

Sea salt and freshly ground black pepper

Optional

Unwaxed lime wedges to serve

* coeliacs please use gluten-free ingredients

Preheat the oven to 200°C/400°F/Gas mark 6.

Place the fish on a non-stick baking tray. In a small bowl, mix the rosemary with the oil, garlic, breadcrumbs, salt and pepper and spread the mixture over the top of each fish steak. Bake in the oven for about 20 minutes until the crumbs are golden and the fish is opaque and cooked through.

Serve immediately with lime wedges.

Stuffed Sardines with Pine Nuts and Spinach

Fresh sardines are quick to cook and much under-valued in England, whereas in Spain and Portugal they are a traditional staple of the diet. They are usually spiced up with plenty of chilli sauce and moistened with fresh aromatic lemons. Here they have the addition of a fresh and light stuffing.

Serves 2

GF   DF   Q&E

115g/3½oz washed fresh spinach leaves, tough stalks removed
30g/⅓ cup pine nuts, toasted
1 tablespoon chopped flat-leaf parsley
30g/1oz organic butter or dairy-free margarine, in small pieces and softened
Sea salt and freshly ground black pepper
4 fresh sardines, gutted and cleaned (or 2 if they are large)
Cold pressed extra virgin olive oil for drizzling

Optional
Cayenne pepper for dusting
Unwaxed lemon or lime wedges to serve

Cook the spinach in a pan of boiling water until just wilted. Drain and squeeze out as much water as possible from the leaves. Coarsely chop the spinach and transfer to a bowl. Mix in the pine nuts, parsley, butter or margarine and season to taste with salt and pepper.

Place the sardines on a non-stick baking tray, making sure that they don't touch each other. Fill the cavities of the sardines with the mixture and lightly close up the fish. Drizzle the fish with oil and dust with cayenne. Grill (broil) the sardines for about 4 minutes on each side until golden and crispy.

Drain on absorbent kitchen paper and serve with wedges of lemon or lime.

Penne with Trout, Fresh Peas and Lemon

Peas have been found in Bronze Age settlements and were cultivated by the ancient Greeks and Romans. In medieval Britain, dried peas were the staple fare, but it was not until the 17th century that fresh peas were introduced from Italy and became fashionable. Now in the 21st century, they are canned and frozen! I hope this Italian-style recipe will revive the fashion for fresh peas.

Serves 4 (double the quantities for the menu on page 297)

GF DF RF

---

2 fresh trout (about 525g/1lb 3oz) – get the fishmonger to gut (clean) them and remove the heads and tails
Sea salt and freshly ground black pepper
255g/10oz pack wheat-free penne*
225g/2 scant cups fresh peas
4 heaped tablespoons coarsely chopped fresh mint leaves
20g/¾oz fresh flat-leaf parsley, coarsely chopped
5 tablespoons fat-free French dressing or cold pressed extra virgin olive oil
Finely grated rind and juice of 1 unwaxed lemon
Minced chilli in oil, according to taste

---

* coeliacs please use gluten-free ingredients

Put a large pan of salted water on to boil. Meanwhile, wash the trout and season the skin with salt and pepper. You can cook the trout on a dish in the microwave until cooked through and opaque, but the time will depend on the size of each fish. Alternatively, steam, poach or grill (broil) the fish. I like to wrap them up loosely in foil with a generous sprinkling of water and bake them for about 20 minutes at 200°C/400°F/Gas mark 6.

Leave the trout to cool before removing the skin from both sides. Carefully lift the flesh off the bones and transfer to a plate. Pick out any remaining bones and then repeat with the underside.

When the pan of water has come to the boil, add the pasta and cook according to the instructions on the pack, or until al dente. Drain and refresh under cold water. Use the same pan to boil enough water to cook the peas in. Cook the peas for 3 minutes, or until tender, then drain and refresh with cold water.

Break the trout into fork-sized pieces, transfer to a pasta bowl and add the mint and parsley. Next, add the pasta and pour in the dressing, lemon rind and juice, season well and add the peas and chilli to taste. Toss the pasta salad carefully so that the trout doesn't break up and serve at room temperature, or keep chilled until needed.

Smoked Trout and Guacamole Rolls

This is a great idea for picnics or a lunch box, and you can also fill the rolls with freshly poached or grilled (broiled) trout. If you would like to try this, then let the cooked trout cool, so that you can handle it. Remove the head, skin and tail and lift off the top fillets. Remove the spine and little bones and you will get to the bottom fillets. Fill the rolls with the trout fillets while still warm and serve with a mixed salad. One small trout will serve 2 people in this way. This recipe uses the famous wild Scottish trout, which is lovingly smoked and then sent all over the world.

GF   DF   Q&E

Serves 4

Guacamole

1 tomato, peeled
1 ripe avocado, preferably Fuerte
Juice of 1 small lime
2 spring onions (scallions), chopped
1 small garlic clove, chopped
15g/½oz fresh coriander (cilantro), trimmed and chopped
1 fresh red medium–hot chilli, chopped (seeds removed if too hot)
Sea salt and freshly ground black pepper

Filling and rolls

1 pack of 2 prepared wild Scottish smoked trout fillets, split into 4 pieces
4 warm wheat-free bread rolls* (see page 304 for stockist), sliced across but not all the way through

* coeliacs please use gluten-free ingredients

First make the guacamole. Cut the tomato into quarters, remove the pith and seeds and discard. Put the tomato flesh into a food processor or blender. Cut the avocado in half, and remove the stone. Scoop the flesh out of the shell and add it to the tomatoes. Add the lime, onions, garlic, coriander (cilantro) and chilli and process until almost smooth, and then scrape into a bowl and season to taste with salt and pepper.

Transfer the guacamole into a bowl and cover with clingfilm (plastic wrap) or a tight-fitting lid and chill for 1 hour before serving.

To assemble the recipe, just heap the guacamole filling into the roll and gently rest the smoked trout on the top. Close the roll and serve with a mixed salad and herbs.

Thai Fish Cakes with Lime Dipping Sauce

My husband loves fish cakes, but for years I couldn't have them because they were always full of potatoes and butter, and covered with breadcrumbs – not ideal for those of us with food intolerances! My version is much healthier and lighter, too. You can make the fish cakes and the sauce in advance, but keep them covered and chilled until needed later in the day.

GF **DF**

Serves 4 as a main course, 8 as an appetizer

Fish cakes

455g/1lb haddock or any other white fish, skinned and cut into chunks

1 garlic clove, crushed

1cm/½in piece root ginger, coarsely grated

15g/½oz fresh coriander (cilantro), coarsely chopped

Grated rind of 1 unwaxed lime

½ red chilli, seeded and finely chopped

½ small red pepper (bell pepper), seeded and coarsely chopped

Sea salt and freshly ground black pepper

30g/¼ cup sesame seeds

2 tablespoons wheat-free flour mix* lightly seasoned with a little salt and pepper

2 tablespoons cold pressed extra virgin olive oil

Dipping sauce

2 spring onions (scallions), heavily trimmed and finely chopped

1 tablespoon cold pressed sunflower oil

Juice of 1 lime

1 tablespoon saké (rice wine)

2 tablespoons soy sauce*

½ red chilli, seeded and finely chopped

2 teaspoons runny honey

2 teaspoons chopped fresh coriander (cilantro) leaves

Optional

Little chillies and sprigs of coriander (cilantro) to decorate

* coeliacs please use gluten-free ingredients

Briefly blend together the fish cake ingredients, except the seasoned flour and oil, in a food processor so that the mixture is minced but not a purée. Transfer it to a bowl and shape the fish cake mixture into 16 small, flattish rounds.

To make the dipping sauce, combine all the ingredients together in a bowl and then transfer to a little serving dish until needed.

Put the seasoned flour on a plate and then coat the fish cakes with it. Heat the oil in a non-stick frying pan (skillet) over high heat and fry the fish cakes until golden on each side. They will only take about 2 minutes on each side. Drain them on absorbent kitchen paper and then transfer to a warm serving dish and serve immediately with the dipping sauce. For a main course, serve these fish cakes accompanied by a bowl of crispy stir-fried vegetables.

Crispy Scallops with Pak Choi

Scallops are expensive but you don't need many for this very light and summery main course. You can serve it with other oriental dishes and a bowl of fragrant steamed rice.

Serves 2

GF DF RF Q&E

Dipping sauce
1½ tablespoons saké (rice wine)
1½ tablespoons soy sauce*
2 teaspoons runny honey
½ red chilli, seeded and finely sliced
1 spring onion (scallion), finely sliced
1 teaspoon finely grated root ginger
2 teaspoons finely chopped fresh coriander (cilantro) leaves

Scallops
15g/2 tablespoons wheat-free flour mix*
Freshly ground black pepper
Pinch of cayenne pepper
1 tablespoon cold pressed extra virgin olive oil and a little extra for frying the scallops
4 baby pak choi, quartered
1 tablespoon Thai fish sauce*
Freshly ground black pepper
8 large scallops

* coeliacs please use gluten-free ingredients

First make the dipping sauce: mix the saké, soy sauce, honey, chilli, spring onion (scallion) and ginger in a small pan and cook for 1 minute over a medium heat, transfer to a small serving bowl, add the coriander (cilantro) and reserve until needed.

Now prepare the scallops. Sift the flour, pepper and cayenne onto a plate. Heat 1 tablespoon of oil in a wok and stir-fry the pak choi for a few minutes so that it wilts slightly. Add the Thai fish sauce and black pepper and cook for another couple of minutes. Arrange the pak choi on a serving dish and keep hot.

Dip the scallops in enough of the flour mixture to coat them. Preheat a non-stick frying pan (skillet) until it is very hot, add a drizzle of oil and then fry the scallops until golden. Do not over-cook the scallops, a couple of minutes should do. Drain them on absorbent kitchen paper. Arrange the scallops on top of the pak choi and serve immediately with the dipping sauce.

Spiced Tuna on Noodles

If you wish, you can omit the rice noodles and replace them with plenty of coarsely grated raw carrots and courgettes (zucchini) – these should be stir-fried with the bean sprouts.

Serves 4

| GF | DF | RF | Q&E |

Marinade

4 spring onions (scallions), heavily trimmed and finely sliced

2 heaped teaspoons coarsely chopped fresh root ginger

1 garlic clove, crushed

2 tablespoons cold pressed extra virgin olive oil

3 tablespoons soy sauce*

2 tablespoons saké (rice wine)

2 tablespoons rice wine vinegar

1 tablespoon runny honey

½ red chilli, finely chopped (remove seeds if too hot)

Tuna and noodles

680g/1½lbs skinless tuna steak

125g/4½oz straight fine rice noodles

2 tablespoons cold pressed extra virgin olive oil

255g/9oz pack fresh bean sprouts

20g/¾oz torn fresh coriander (cilantro) leaves, and an extra 7g/¼oz serving

Optional

Chilli sauce* or minced chilli in oil according to taste

* coeliacs please use gluten-free ingredients

The Big Book of Wheat-Free Cooking

First make the marinade. Place all the ingredients together in a bowl, heat a wok over a high heat for a few seconds and then pour in the marinade. Cook for about a minute to release the flavours. Transfer the marinade to a dish in which you will be able to marinate the tuna strips and leave the mixture to cool.

Cut the tuna into thin strips about 12mm/½in wide, place them in the cold marinade, cover the dish and chill for 15 minutes. Now turn the strips of tuna over and marinate for another 15 minutes.

Pour boiling water on to the noodles in a bowl, to soften them – about 3 minutes should do it. Drain them and then heat the oil in the wok over a medium heat and stir-fry the noodles with the bean sprouts, 20g/¾oz coriander (cilantro) and chilli for a couple of minutes. Season to taste with pepper and salt if necessary.

Transfer the noodle mixture to a warm serving dish and keep warm. Heat the wok again over a high heat and quickly fry the fish in the marinade, for about a minute on each side. Try not to break up the tuna. Carefully lay the tuna strips on top of the noodles and pour over the marinade. Sprinkle with extra coriander (cilantro) and serve immediately.

Chargrilled Squid with Herb Dressing

Squid looks so off-putting, but in fact it is quick and easy to cook and not expensive. You can find it frozen all year round in the fishmonger's but do make sure he prepares it for you. You need whole cleaned tubes and the tentacles to be separate.

Serves 4   GF   DF   RF   Q&E

Herb dressing

45g/1½oz flat-leaf parsley leaves

15g/½oz fresh mint leaves

15g/½oz fresh coriander (cilantro) leaves

1 teaspoon each ground cumin and coriander seeds

Finely grated rind and juice of 1 large unwaxed lemon

4 tablespoons cold pressed extra virgin olive oil

2 small chillies, sliced

A pinch of sea salt

Fish

225g/3 cups sliced runner beans (I like diamond-shaped lengths)

Freshly ground black pepper

12–16 small squid, prepared and washed (tentacles separated)

Drizzle of cold pressed extra virgin olive oil

The Big Book of Wheat-Free Cooking

To make the herb dressing, chop the herbs in the food processor but not too finely. Toast the cumin and the coriander seeds in a small, dry, non-stick pan over a medium high heat until they release a strong aroma, and then add to the herbs. Add the grated rind and juice of the lemon, oil, chillies and salt. Blend until finely chopped but not puréed.

Cook the runner beans in boiling water for 3 minutes, then drain and rinse under cold water. Arrange the beans evenly over the serving dish and sprinkle with freshly ground black pepper.

Slit the squid open along one side and, using a sharp knife, mark a tiny crisscross pattern on top. Cook the squid and the tentacles in a drizzle of oil on a preheated chargrill or in a preheated ridged pan for about a minute on each side.

Place the squid in short rows diagonally along the beans. Spoon the herb dressing over the squid and serve immediately. This dish is delicious accompanied by simple salads, such as green leaves and herbs or tomato and cucumber.

Chilled Halibut with Two Salsas

This is such a bright and cheerful summer dish. I much prefer chilled fish to warm – the texture is much firmer and I find the flavours are more concentrated. You can use cheaper seasonal white fish, or fish such as salmon, tuna and swordfish steaks. Serve this dish with a big green salad and some chilled French beans lightly sprinkled with lemon juice and olive oil.

GF DF RF

Serves 4

4 halibut steaks, around 900g/2lb total weight including bone

Juice of ½ a lemon

Sea salt and freshly ground black pepper

4 bay leaves

4 wedges of unwaxed lime to serve and a little fresh parsley to decorate

Herb salsa

1 tablespoon capers* (not in malt vinegar), rinsed in cold water for 10 minutes

3 anchovy fillets, soaked in a saucer of cold water for 10 minutes

6 bottled baby cornichons* (cocktail gherkins) not in malt vinegar, drained

1 garlic clove, crushed

15g/½oz mint leaves

15g/½oz flat-leaf parsley leaves

15g/½oz basil leaves

Juice of ½ a lemon

Approximately 5 tablespoons bottled fat-free French dressing and 2 tablespoons cold pressed extra virgin olive oil

1 teaspoon Dijon mustard*

Sea salt, if needed, and freshly ground black pepper

Pepper salsa

1 tablespoon cold pressed extra virgin olive oil

400g/14oz can chopped tomatoes

1 medium–hot red chilli, finely chopped

15g/½oz oregano leaves, coarsely chopped

1 garlic clove, sliced

1 teaspoon balsamic vinegar

2 small red peppers (bell peppers), seeded and coarsely chopped

Sea salt and freshly ground black pepper

* coeliacs please use gluten-free ingredients

Preheat the oven to 200°C/400°F/Gas mark 6.

Lay the fish on a baking tray, squeeze the lemon juice over, season lightly with salt and pepper, place a bay leaf on top of each steak and cover lightly with foil. Bake in the oven for about 15 minutes. To test if it is cooked, gently push a skewer into the thickest part of the flesh – if it is too firm then it is not ready yet. When it is cooked through, lightly cover the fish with the foil and leave it to cool.

Make the herb salsa. Put the capers, anchovies, cornichons, garlic and herbs into a food processor and whizz until finely chopped. Transfer to a bowl and, by hand, stir in the lemon juice, dressing, olive oil and mustard and season to taste with salt and pepper. Transfer to a container to chill until needed (but serve at room temperature).

Make the pepper (bell pepper) salsa. Heat the olive oil in a saucepan and add the tomatoes, chilli, oregano, garlic, vinegar and peppers. Simmer for about 20 minutes or until the peppers (bell peppers) are cooked through. Cool the mixture before processing in a food processor, whizzing it to the consistency of a chunky purée. Season with salt and freshly ground pepper and transfer to a container to chill until needed.

Once the fish has cooled, carefully remove it from its baking tray and put it on a dish in the refrigerator. To prepare the dish, gently peel off the fish skin, remove the bones and arrange the fillets in a line down the centre of a serving dish. Spoon one salsa down one side and the remaining salsa along the other side and decorate with the lime wedges and parsley. Keep chilled until needed.

Roast Cod with Pineapple Salsa

Fish such as cod often crumbles and breaks up before it is cooked through. A good tip is to season it with a little salt two hours before you cook it, so that the protein in the fish will firm up and it won't fall apart. The unusual combination of cod and pineapple comes from the Caribbean-style idea of mixing fruit with fish. This has a refreshing sweet-and-sour effect.

Serves 6

GF **DF** **RF** **Q&E**

Salsa

1 small pineapple, peeled and the eyes dug out, quartered, core removed and flesh chopped into small pieces
1 tablespoon cold pressed extra virgin olive oil
1 tablespoon runny honey
400g/14oz can chopped tomatoes
4 spring onions (scallions), heavily trimmed and very finely sliced
½ red chilli (any strength), seeded and very finely sliced
Finely grated rind and juice of 1 unwaxed lime
2 tablespoons chopped fresh coriander (cilantro) leaves
Sea salt and freshly ground black pepper
Light sprinkling of cayenne pepper

Fish

6 thick cod steaks or other white fish, must be thick enough to roast, about 900g/2lbs
Juice of 1 lime
Sea salt and freshly ground black pepper
Sprinkling of cayenne pepper

Optional

Unwaxed lime quarters and fresh coriander (cilantro) to decorate

Preheat the oven to 200°C/400°F/Gas mark 6.

Make the salsa. Fry the pineapple in the oil in a non-stick frying pan (skillet), over a medium heat, for about 3 minutes. Pour the honey over the pineapple and keep frying until the pineapple has lovely browned caramelized bits. Shaking the pan and stirring will prevent it burning.

Remove from the heat, transfer to a bowl and stir in all the remaining salsa ingredients. If you are making this in advance, you can leave it to cool, cover it and chill it until needed but serve at room temperature.

About 15 minutes before needed, put the cod steaks into a baking dish, sprinkle with lime juice, black pepper and cayenne pepper; there is no need to salt the fish if you did so earlier to firm it up.

Roast the fish in the oven for 10 minutes or until opaque and just cooked through. Serve the fish on warm plates with a large dollop of salsa. Decorate with lime quarters and fresh coriander (cilantro).

Swordfish Palermo

As the best swordfish is reputed to come from Sicily, I thought a local recipe full of traditional ingredients would be fun; this dish makes a nice change from the designer food so often eaten in trendy restaurants.

   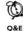

Serves 4

GF   DF   RF   Q&E

---

2 swordfish steaks, about 340g/12oz each
1 tablespoon cold pressed extra virgin olive oil
1 large red onion, finely chopped
2 garlic cloves, crushed
4 anchovy fillets, drained and finely chopped
400g/14oz can chopped tomatoes
1 tablespoon chopped fresh rosemary
1 tablespoon capers* in sherry vinegar, drained
Sea salt and freshly ground black pepper
7g/¼oz fresh flat-leaf parsley, chopped

---

coeliacs please use gluten-free ingredients

Wash the swordfish steaks and pat them dry with absorbent kitchen paper. Heat a non-stick frying pan (skillet) until very hot and then dry-fry the swordfish for a couple of minutes on each side. Remove them from the pan and keep warm. Reduce the heat to medium and then, in the same pan, heat the olive oil and stir in the onions. Cook until soft but not browned. Stir in the garlic, anchovies, tomatoes, rosemary and capers and cook for 20 minutes.

Season to taste with salt and pepper and then return the swordfish steaks to the pan with the sauce and simmer until they are warmed through.

Place on a serving dish and serve immediately, sprinkled with parsley. Divide the steaks into 4 pieces at the table.

Oriental Smoked Salmon

This is the ultimate easy appetizer, which I use all the time. The better quality the salmon, the smoother the taste will be. Cheap, oily salmon on special offer tends to be just that, oily, and tasteless. This recipe is also delicious with wafer-thin slices of extremely fresh raw salmon – my version of sushi!

Serves 4

DF RF Q&E

8 slices of good-quality smoked salmon about 50g/2oz each
⅓ of a 90g/3oz pack pickled ginger* (pink and sliced)

Dressing
1 heaped teaspoon Dijon mustard*
Sea salt and freshly ground black pepper
½ red chilli (any strength), seeded and finely chopped
2 teaspoons runny honey
2 tablespoons pickled ginger vinegar*
7g/¼oz very finely sliced fresh coriander (cilantro) leaves
2 tablespoons cold pressed sunflower oil

* coeliacs please use gluten-free ingredients

Arrange the smoked salmon on a serving plate and carefully lay the pickled ginger slices over it.

To make the dressing, mix all the ingredients together in the given order in a bowl. Sprinkle the dressing all over the salmon and ginger. Serve immediately or cover and chill until needed.

Three Star Tostaditas

The following three recipes are quick and easy, and with no cooking needed, they are ideal as appetizers for a barbecue while everything else is charring nicely over the charcoal. Tostaditas are also brilliant for drinks parties in the summer. Please note that while packs of corn chips may say 100% corn and therefore be gluten-free, the coating may not be, so check the label carefully.

The three different toppings should be enough for 10–16 people. Arrange the three types of Nachips together on a big dish or several smaller ones and keep chilled until served. Do not assemble more than a couple of hours in advance otherwise they may go soggy.

Tostaditas with guacamole and prawns (shrimp)

Makes about 20

GF DF

200g/7oz king prawns (jumbo shrimp)
Juice of 1 lime
Pinch of cayenne pepper
½ garlic clove, crushed
200g/7oz pack pure corn Nachips* or similar fried corn wafers* or Nachos* (for all 3 toppings)

Guacamole

2 tomatoes, peeled, halved and seeded
2 ripe avocados, preferably Fuerte
Juice of 1 lime
1 spring onion (scallion), heavily trimmed then chopped
1 garlic clove, chopped
15g/½oz fresh coriander (cilantro), chopped
1 fresh red medium–hot chilli, chopped (seeds removed for a milder taste)
Sea salt and freshly ground black pepper

coeliacs please use gluten-free ingredients

First marinate the prawns (shrimp). In a bowl mix together the lime juice, cayenne and garlic and marinate the prawns (shrimp) for at least 1 hour, keeping them chilled until needed.

Now make the guacamole. Place the tomato halves in a food processor. Cut the avocados in half and remove the stones. Scoop the flesh out of the shells and place it with the tomatoes. Add the lime juice, onion, garlic, coriander (cilantro) and chilli and process until almost smooth, then scrape into a bowl and season to taste with salt and pepper.

Cover with clingfilm (plastic wrap), or a tight-fitting lid, and chill for 1 hour before serving. To assemble this dish, just place a dollop of guacamole on to each Nachip, probably about 20, top with a prawn (shrimp) and sprinkle with coriander (cilantro).

Tostaditas with sweetcorn and pepper (bell pepper)

Makes about 16

GF DF V

2 red peppers (bell peppers), halved and seeded
A little cold pressed virgin olive oil
I teaspoon chopped fresh rosemary
300g/10½oz jar sweetcorn relish*
7g/¼oz fresh parsley, chopped

coeliacs please use gluten-free ingredients

Brush the peppers (bell peppers) with oil and sprinkle with rosemary. Grill (broil) them until black patches appear on the skin and then peel off the skin using a sharp knife. Cut the pepper (bell pepper) into attractive slithers. Spoon dollops of sweetcorn relish on to at least 16 Nachips, decorate with the peppers and sprinkle with a little chopped parsley.

Tostaditas with crab and mango

Makes about 14

GF DF

150g/5oz fresh crab meat
Good squeeze of lime juice
A little chilli sauce* or minced chilli in oil
Sea salt and freshly ground black pepper
I spring onion (scallion), finely chopped
About ½ a ripe mango, peeled and cut into attractive slithers or chunks
15 fresh basil leaves for decoration

coeliacs please use gluten-free ingredients

Mix the crab meat with the lime juice, chilli, seasoning and onion in a bowl. Spoon dollops of the mixture on to about 14 Nachips and decorate each one with a little mango and a basil leaf.

Meat, Poultry and Game ...

Beef Casserole with Dijon Croûtons

You can swap the chestnuts in this recipe for mushrooms if you prefer, or you can use pickled walnuts* as another delicious alternative. You can freeze the casserole in advance, defrost it and then reheat it with the prepared croûtons. This is a great dish for large gatherings – hence the number of servings – as it is delicious, simple and allows the chef plenty of free time to enjoy the party.

Serves 12

GF   DF

---

4 tablespoons cold pressed extra virgin olive oil

2 very large onions, thinly sliced

1.9kg/4lb 4oz shin beef, trimmed, cut into generous bite-size pieces and dipped into 3 heaped tablespoons well seasoned wheat-free flour mix*

2 large celery sticks, tough threads removed, chopped

2 large carrots, peeled and finely chopped

440ml/1 large can ale or stout* (coeliacs could also use red wine)

1 heaped teaspoon unrefined dark soft brown sugar

1 heaped tablespoon tomato purée (paste)

1 tablespoon Worcestershire sauce*

2 sachets bouquet garni

Sea salt and freshly ground black pepper

340g/3 cups canned peeled cooked chestnuts, drained (or vacuum packed or frozen is fine)

500ml/2 cups allergy-free vegetable, chicken or beef stock (bouillon)

Dijon croûtons

1 heaped tablespoon soft organic butter or dairy-free margarine

1 heaped tablespoon Dijon mustard*

2 teaspoons dried thyme leaves

6 Dietary Specials sweet gluten-free white breakfast rolls, halved horizontally (you will need 2 packets) (see page 307 for stockist)

One very large heatproof casserole with a lid (use a shallow and wide or long one rather than a smaller very deep casserole otherwise you won't be able to arrange the croûtons on top)

---

* *coeliacs please use gluten-free ingredients*

Preheat the oven to 180°C/350°F/Gas mark 4.

Heat 2 tablespoons of the oil in the casserole dish, add the onions and fry until softened and tinged with gold. Remove the onions to a plate and keep to one side. Add the remaining oil to the casserole, add the beef and briefly sauté until it is sealed and browned. Return the onions to the casserole and add the celery, carrot, ale or stout, sugar, tomato purée (paste), Worcestershire sauce and bouquet garni. Top up the casserole with 500ml/2 cups of filtered water, season with salt and pepper, cover the casserole and bring to boiling point. Immediately transfer the casserole to the oven and cook for 2 hours.

Ten minutes before the end of cooking time, make the croûtons. Mix the butter or margarine in a little bowl with the mustard and thyme and season with salt and pepper. Spread each half of each roll with the mixture.

Remove the casserole from the oven, stir in the chestnuts and arrange the croûtons over the top. Return the casserole to the oven and bake, uncovered, for about 20–30 minutes until the croûtons are golden. Serve the casserole before the croûtons become soggy.

Steak with Parmesan and Mushrooms

This dish can be made in the morning for a special dinner, leaving you more time to relax before your guests arrive. The Smoked Salmon and Crab Timbales on page 44 can also be made in advance, which makes the two recipes a natural choice for an impressive menu. Finish the meal with the Chestnut Parfait on page 206, which you can make up to 2 days in advance, and you will have even more energy to devote to having fun!

GF   **DF**   **Q&E**

Serves 4

680g/1½lbs middle cut beef fillet

Crushed black peppercorns

2 tablespoons olive oil

1 small onion, finely chopped

1 garlic clove, crushed

255g/9oz mixed mushrooms (wild and cultivated), sliced

2 tablespoons sherry or Madeira

Sea salt and freshly ground black pepper

Freshly grated nutmeg

1 tablespoon crème fraîche or dairy-free Tofutti Sour Supreme (see page 305 for stockist)

1 organic free-range egg yolk

1 tablespoon chopped fresh parsley

2 tablespoons freshly grated Parmesan or Florentino Parmazano (see page 306 for stockist)

Trim the fillet and roll in the crushed black peppercorns. Warm 1 tablespoon of the oil in a frying pan (skillet) and sauté the meat until it is browned on all sides – this will take about 10 minutes if you like it medium-rare. Leave it to cool on a wire rack over a plate.

Add the remaining oil to the pan, add the onion and cook gently until soft. Stir in the garlic and mushrooms. Increase the heat and cook for a couple of minutes before adding the sherry. Cook for about 5 minutes until the mushrooms are cooked and the liquid has been absorbed. Transfer the mixture to a bowl, season with salt, pepper and nutmeg and leave to cool.

When the mixture is cold, stir in the crème fraîche or Sour Supreme, egg yolk and parsley and chill. Wrap the meat in a tight roll of clingfilm (plastic wrap) and chill until 15 minutes before eating.

Preheat the oven to 200°C/400°F/Gas mark 6.

Unwrap the beef and cut into 4 even-sized pieces. Place them on a lightly greased baking tray or ovenproof dish. Spoon the mushroom mixture onto each steak, flatten slightly and sprinkle with the cheese. Cook, uncovered, for about 8 minutes until the tops are golden and bubbling.

Serve immediately with vegetables and new potatoes, or salad and sauté potatoes or French fries. I also love having the choice of horseradish sauce or mustard with the steak but check the labels to ensure that they don't contain wheat or gluten.

Conchiglie with Salami, Fennel and Tomatoes

I like this dish in the summer with a big salad and a plate of roast sweet peppers. Parma ham can be used instead of salami or bacon if you prefer.

Serves 4–6

GF   DF   Q&E

370g/12oz packet gluten-free pasta shells* (any brand)
Sea salt
2 tablespoons cold pressed extra virgin olive oil
2 small fennel bulbs, trimmed and finely sliced
1 small red onion, finely sliced
1kg/2¼lb fresh ripe vine tomatoes, peeled, seeded and chopped or 3 x 400g/14oz cans chopped tomatoes
2 heaped tablespoons tomato purée (paste)
15g/½oz fresh basil leaves, shredded
155g/5½oz packet rindless salami slices* (check label for starch)
Freshly ground black pepper
1 tablespoon lemon juice

Optional
Extra basil to garnish and freshly grated pecorino cheese or dairy-free Florentino Parmazano (see page 306 for stockist)

* coeliacs please use gluten-free ingredients

Bring a pan of salted water to the boil, cook the pasta until softened, stirring and separating the pasta from time to time. Drain the pasta and refresh with cold water. Refill the pan with salted water, bring it to the boil and cook the pasta until soft, stirring from time to time. (This method prevents the pasta becoming sticky.)

Meanwhile, heat the oil in a pan, add the fennel and onions and sauté until they are tinged with gold and soft. Stir in the tomatoes, tomato purée (paste), shredded basil and salami and simmer until the vegetables are cooked. Season to taste with salt, pepper and lemon juice.

Drain the pasta, transfer to a warm serving bowl, toss in the sauce and serve immediately, with or without the grated cheese.

Spaghetti with Ham and Flageolet Bean Sauce

I made this dish with some of the leftover roast Christmas ham; it is rustic and strong flavoured, which is ideal in the middle of winter. I serve it as a first course, followed by a huge mixed salad with roasted vegetables and a selection of cheeses but you can of course serve it as a main course.

GF   DF   Q&E

Serves 3 as a main course or 4 as an appetizer

340g/12oz wheat-free spaghetti* (any brand)
Sea salt
4 tablespoons cold pressed extra virgin olive oil
170g/6oz diced roast ham or if pre-sliced cut into thin strips, all fat removed
2 garlic cloves, crushed
1 heaped tablespoon chopped fresh parsley
1 tablespoon chopped fresh sage leaves
2 teaspoons finely chopped rosemary
A sprinkling of dried chilli flakes
400g/14oz can flageolet beans, drained
Sea salt and freshly ground black pepper
2 tablespoons dry white wine
4 heaped tablespoons freshly grated pecorino cheese or dairy-free Florentino Parmazano, plus extra if desired (see page 306 for stockist)

* coeliacs please use gluten-free ingredients

Bring a pan of salted water to the boil, add the spaghetti and cook until softened, stirring and separating the pasta from time to time. Drain the pasta and refresh with cold water. Refill the pan with salted water, bring it to the boil and cook the pasta until soft, stirring from time to time. (This method prevents the pasta becoming sticky.)

Heat half the oil in a pan, add the ham, garlic, herbs and chilli and sauté for about 3 minutes. Add the remaining oil, beans, seasoning and wine and cook for about 3 minutes, stirring occasionally.

Drain the pasta, transfer to a warm serving bowl and toss with the ham sauce and the cheese. Adjust the seasoning and serve.

Italian Roast Partridge

The traditional season for partridge is from 1 September to 1 February. As with all seasonal things, they are more expensive at the beginning of the season when they tend to be young and tender. I serve this dish with either Cranberry and Pistachio Rice or Parmesan and Olive Oil Mash (see pages 191 and 194) as both can be prepared in advance and kept warm until you are ready to serve the partridges.

Serves 4–5 (double the ingredients for the Christmas eve menu on page 295)

GF

4 or 5 prepared partridges, rinsed clean under cold running water

Sea salt and freshly ground black pepper

200g/scant cup organic mascarpone cheese

1 heaped teaspoon dried oregano leaves

4 tablespoons chopped fresh parsley

1 teaspoon finely chopped rosemary

8–10 slices rindless smoked back bacon

4–5 bay leaves

A drizzle of cold pressed extra virgin olive oil

250ml/1 cup red wine

250ml/1 cup allergy-free chicken stock (bouillon)

1 tablespoon pure cornflour (cornstarch)

A knob of organic butter

Preheat the oven to 200°C/400°F/Gas mark 6.

Put the partridges on a clean board and season the cavities with a little salt and pepper. In a bowl, mix the cheese and chopped herbs and season to taste.

Carefully ease and lift up the skin of each bird without tearing it so that you can push in the cheese stuffing. Using your hands, gently spread and shape the stuffing under the skin so that the birds look nice and rounded.

Wrap each partridge in two slices of bacon and set each one on a bay leaf in a roasting pan. Drizzle the birds with the oil, pour in the wine and stock (bouillon) and roast in the oven for about 35 minutes. If you pierce the thighs with a sharp knife the juices should run clear when the birds are cooked through.

Transfer the partridges onto hot plates. Mix the cornflour (cornstarch) with 2 tablespoons of cold filtered water and stir it into the pan juices. Bring the juices to the boil over high heat, stirring and scraping the pan; add more liquid if necessary and cook until you have a thick sauce. Remove from the heat, stir in the knob of butter and adjust the seasoning if necessary. Spoon the sauce over each partridge and serve immediately.

Buckwheat Galettes with Ham and Cheese

I first made this recipe with ham and leftover Stilton at Christmas but you can make it with Emmental cheese or with a dairy-free grated Cheddar-style hard cheese. Serve the galettes with mixed salad leaves and fresh herbs, drizzled with a little oil and balsamic vinegar.

GF   DF

Makes 6–8 large pancakes

60g/scant ½ cup organic buckwheat flour

60g/scant ½ cup organic rice flour

2 large organic free-range eggs

4 tablespoons cold pressed extra virgin olive oil

Fine salt and freshly ground black pepper

55g/2oz organic butter or dairy-free margarine

6–8 thin slices cooked ham, fat removed

310g/11oz piece organic Stilton, crumbled, Emmental, coarsely grated or dairy-free Cheddar-style cheese, grated (see page 305 for stockist)

25.5cm/10in non-stick frying pan (skillet)

The Big Book of Wheat-Free Cooking

Put the flours, eggs, 2 tablespoons of the oil and salt in a food processor and blend with 150ml/½ cup cold filtered water. Process until smooth and then add the same quantity of water again and blend until well mixed. Allow the batter to rest for 30 minutes.

Melt 15g/½oz of the butter or margarine in small pan with the remaining oil. Meanwhile, heat the frying pan (skillet) until hot but not smoking. Use a little of the melted butter and oil mixture to grease the pan before making each pancake. Ladle in and swirl around enough batter to cover the base of the pan and cook the pancake until golden, then flip over and cook the other side. Layer each galette between sheets of non-stick baking parchment (wax paper) until all the batter is used.

Lay each galette flat and cover with a slice of ham and a layer of crumbled or grated cheese. Season with pepper and fold in half.

Melt the remaining butter in the pancake pan and fry two galettes at a time until they are crisp on both sides and the cheese has melted on the inside. This won't take more than a few minutes on each side so be warned – if you cook them for too long the cheese seems to disappear!

Chicken with Olives and Potatoes

This delicious Mediterranean-style dish is perfect for the summer and the quantities can easily be doubled if you are having lots of friends round for an alfresco lunch.

The chicken only needs a big bowl of mixed salad with plenty of basil and a drizzle of oil to accompany it.

GF   DF   RF

Serves about 8

Large family-sized (2.75–3kg/6–6½lb) organic roasting chicken, any string, fat or giblets removed and discarded
Cold pressed extra virgin olive oil
1 tablespoon paprika
Sea salt and freshly ground black pepper
36 large pitted black olives in oil not vinegar, drained
1kg/2¼lb potatoes, scrubbed clean and cut lengthways into thin slices

Optional
Fresh basil leaves and unwaxed lemon wedges to serve

Preheat the oven to 200°C/400°F/Gas mark 6.

Rub the chicken all over with a little oil and sprinkle it evenly with the paprika. Season inside the bird with salt and pepper and place it in a large baking/roasting tin (pan). Drizzle oil around the chicken and throw in the olives and potatoes. Season everything with salt and pepper, and drizzle with a little more oil.

Roast in the oven for about 55 minutes, then baste the chicken and turn all the potatoes and olives over so that they cook evenly. Cook for a further 50 minutes.

Transfer the chicken to a large hot serving dish, surround the bird with the potatoes and olives and scatter with basil and lemon wedges.

To serve four people: halve the ingredients and cook the smaller chicken in the same way – give it about 35 minutes before basting the bird and turning the potatoes then cook for about 25 minutes more.

Italian Shepherd's Pie

This recipe is much faster to make than a traditional shepherd's pie, as the topping comes ready-prepared. You can make double the quantity and freeze one for an instant meal.

Serves 4

GF   DF   Q&E

1 large onion, finely chopped
1 tablespoon cold pressed extra virgin olive oil
500g/1lb 2oz pack good quality minced (ground) beef
1 large thick carrot, finely chopped
500g/1lb 2oz jar Dolmio sauce for Bolognese or other brands of tomato sauce*
Sea salt and freshly ground black pepper
500g/1lb 2oz ready-made pure corn polenta
55g/2oz Parmesan, coarsely grated or dairy-free grated Florentino Parmazano (see page 306 for stockist)

Optional
Red wine or filtered water if the mixture becomes dry

* coeliacs please use gluten-free ingredients

Fry the onions in the oil until softened, stir in the meat and cook for about 5 minutes until well browned. Stir in the carrots and tomato sauce, season with salt and pepper and simmer until the vegetables and meat are tender. You can add some red wine or filtered water if the mixture becomes too dry.

Cut the polenta into about 16 slices. Tip the meat mixture into an ovenproof serving dish and flatten the surface. Arrange the polenta in overlapping slices all over the top. Sprinkle with the cheese and grill (broil) for about 10–15 minutes until the polenta is hot and the cheese is melted and tinged with brown.

Traditional Lasagne

Lasagne freezes beautifully, which makes it ideal for easy entertaining. Thaw it, bake it for about 20 minutes in a hot oven until bubbling and serve with a large green salad.

GF **DF**

Serves 8

8–10 sheets Orgran gluten-free instant lasagne (see page 305 for stockist)

30g/1oz Parmesan, finely grated or dairy-free Florentino Parmazano (see page 306 for stockist)

Meat sauce

4 tablespoons cold pressed extra virgin olive oil

4 strips rindless back bacon, cut into thin slices

1 large onion, very finely chopped

680g/1½lbs good quality minced (ground) beef

225g/8oz chicken livers, picked over to remove any fat or sinew, then rinsed with cold water and chopped

2 large carrots, finely diced

2 sticks celery, finely diced

2 garlic cloves, crushed

3 heaped tablespoons tomato purée (paste)

1 heaped teaspoon unrefined golden granulated sugar

Sea salt and freshly ground black pepper

1 heaped teaspoon dried oregano

310ml/1¼ cups red wine

310ml/1¼ cups allergy-free beef, vegetable or chicken stock (bouillon)

Cheese sauce

55g/2oz organic butter or dairy-free margarine

30g/1oz wheat-free flour mix* mixed with 30g/1oz pure cornflour (cornstarch)

1 heaped teaspoon mustard*

1 litre/4 cups organic milk or organic unsweetened dairy-free milk

115g/4oz grated organic mature hard cheese or Redwood dairy-free Cheddar-style grated cheese (see page 305 for stockist)

Sea salt and freshly ground black pepper

Freshly grated nutmeg

* coeliacs please use gluten-free ingredients

Preheat the oven to 180°C/350°F/Gas mark 4.

Make the meat sauce first. Heat the oil in a large non-stick pan, add the bacon and cook until tinged with gold. Add the onions and cook until they have softened. Stir in the minced beef, chicken livers, carrots, celery and garlic and cook for a couple of minutes. Stir in the tomato purée (paste), sugar, salt, pepper and herbs. Add the wine and stock (bouillon) and simmer at bubbling point for about an hour, stirring occasionally.

Three quarters of the way through the cooking time, make the cheese sauce. Melt the butter in a saucepan over low heat and stir in the flour and cornflour (cornstarch). Cook gently for 1 minute and stir in the mustard. Gradually stir in the milk a little at a time and beat until you have a runny, smooth sauce. Bring to the boil, stir in the cheese and remove from the heat. Season to taste with salt, pepper and nutmeg.

Spread about one third of the meat mixture over the base of a large ovenproof serving dish. Cover with about 4 or 5 sheets of lasagne and spoon and spread half the cheese sauce over the top. Cover with another third of the meat, repeat the layer of pasta, cover this with the remaining meat and top with the remaining cheese sauce. Sprinkle with the grated Parmesan or Parmazano and bake for about 45 minutes until the lasagne feels soft in the centre.

Pastitsio

This Greek dish is easier to make than Moussaka, as it uses macaroni as the topping rather than having to fry endless aubergines (eggplant).

Serves 4–6

GF   DF

2 tablespoons extra virgin olive oil

1 large onion, finely chopped

2 garlic cloves, crushed

500g/1lb 2oz good quality minced (ground) lamb

2 tablespoons tomato purée (paste)

400g/14oz can chopped tomatoes

1 teaspoon dried thyme

200ml/¾ cup hot allergy-free beef, chicken or vegetable stock (bouillon)

Sea salt and freshly ground black pepper

Sauce and topping

30g/1oz organic butter or dairy-free margarine

30g/1oz wheat-free flour mix*

310ml/1¼ cups organic milk or organic unsweetened dairy-free soya milk

250ml/1 cup single (light) cream or Provamel dairy-free Soya Dream

1 large organic free-range egg, beaten

255g/9oz wheat-free macaroni or pasta tubes* (any brand)

55g/2oz organic mature Cheddar, grated, or dairy-free Redwoods grated Cheddar-style cheese (see page 305 for stockist)

* coeliacs please use gluten-free ingredients

Preheat the oven to 180°C/350°F/Gas mark 4.

Heat the oil in a large pan, add the onion and cook until softened. Stir in the garlic. Add the lamb and fry over high heat for about 3 minutes until browned all over. Stir in the tomato purée (paste) and cook for 1–2 minutes. Stir in the tomatoes, thyme and stock (bouillon) and season with salt and pepper. Reduce the heat and simmer at bubbling point for about 35 minutes.

Meanwhile, cook the pasta in a pan of salted, boiling water until softened, stirring and separating the pasta from time to time. Drain the pasta and refresh with cold water. Refill the pan with salted water, bring it to the boil and cook the pasta until soft, stirring from time to time. (This method prevents the pasta becoming sticky.)

While the pasta is cooking, make the sauce. Melt the butter or margarine in a non-stick pan, stir in the flour and cook gently for a minute before gradually beating in the milk. Stir continuously until the sauce is thick and smooth and reaches boiling point. Remove from the heat and stir in the cream or Soya Dream and the beaten egg. Season with salt and pepper and set aside.

Drain the pasta and spread half of it over the base of an ovenproof serving dish. Cover with the meat and top with the remaining pasta. Pour the sauce over and sprinkle with the grated cheese.

Bake in the oven for about 25 minutes and serve when golden and bubbling.

Chicken Kebabs with Quinoa Couscous

I was delightfully surprised the first time that I cooked quinoa this way – it was so nutty and had a delicious texture, just like couscous. I now use quinoa whenever couscous is called for.

Serves 2

GF **DF**

Quinoa couscous

85g/½ cup quinoa

1 tablespoon extra virgin olive oil

½ small red onion, finely chopped

1 small sweet orange pepper (bell pepper), seeded and finely chopped

1 small sweet green pepper (bell pepper), seeded and finely chopped

1 garlic clove, finely chopped

1 teaspoon dried mixed herbs

500ml/2 cups water or allergy-free vegetable stock (bouillon)

A pinch of cayenne pepper

2 tablespoons chopped fresh parsley

Kebabs

2 small, skinless organic chicken breasts, cut into 10 bite-size pieces

2 large vine tomatoes, quartered

2 large field mushrooms, peeled and quartered

Cold pressed extra virgin olive oil for drizzling

A sprinkling of dried oregano leaves

Fine salt and freshly ground black pepper

2 long bamboo or metal skewers

Soak the quinoa in a bowl of cold water. Meanwhile, heat the oil in a pan, add the onion and cook gently until softened. Drain and rinse the quinoa. Add the peppers, garlic and mixed herbs to the onions and cook for 3 minutes. Add the water or stock (bouillon) and bring to the boil. Stir in the quinoa and cayenne pepper and simmer for about 30 minutes until the liquid is absorbed.

Meanwhile, put the kebabs together. Slide the chicken pieces, tomato quarters and mushroom quarters onto the skewers until you have used up all the ingredients. I suggest starting and finishing with the chicken. Drizzle all the ingredients generously with oil and sprinkle with the oregano, salt and pepper. About 5 minutes before the quinoa is cooked, grill (broil) the kebabs for about 5 minutes on each side until the chicken is cooked through and the vegetables have softened and are hot.

Let the quinoa couscous sit for about 5 minutes before fluffing it up with a fork. Season the quinoa with salt and pepper and sprinkle with parsley. Serve the kebabs on a bed of steaming hot quinoa couscous.

Braised Spiced Lamb Shanks

The lamb shank is the skinny part of the leg and because this region contains lots of connective tissue it needs long, slow cooking. The spice flavours in this recipe are well balanced but if you prefer stronger flavours, you can add more. If possible, start marinating the lamb in the refrigerator one or two days before cooking.

This dish is fabulous served with saffron-flavoured mashed potatoes.

Serves 4–6

GF   DF

Marinade

½ teaspoon each of ground ginger, mace, allspice, cumin, coriander, cinnamon and cloves
1 tablespoon cold pressed extra virgin olive oil
750ml/3 cups red wine
1 onion, sliced
2 garlic cloves, crushed
Parsley stalks
2 bay leaves
1 large strip of unwaxed orange peel
Freshly ground black pepper

Lamb

4–6 lamb shanks
3 tablespoons cold pressed extra virgin olive oil
1 onion, finely chopped
2 large carrots, diced
2 celery sticks, diced
2 large garlic cloves, crushed
560ml/2¼ cups strong allergy-free vegetable stock (bouillon)
2 bay leaves
Sea salt and freshly ground black pepper
3 tablespoons pure cornflour (cornstarch) dissolved in 3 tablespoons cold filtered water
Finely chopped fresh parsley to serve

Dry fry all the spices for the marinade in a non-stick frying pan (skillet), over medium heat, until the spices are smoking and aromatic – this should take less than a minute. Remove from the heat. Mix the fried spices and the remaining marinade ingredients together in a deep, ovenproof serving dish and add the lamb. Cover and refrigerate for 24 hours, turning occasionally.

Preheat the oven to 170°C/325°F/Gas mark 3.

Begin cooking about 2½ hours before serving the meal. Heat 2 tablespoons of oil in a large oven- and flame-proof casserole over medium heat. Add the onion, carrot and celery and cook slowly until golden, then stir in the garlic and cook for 1 minute. Transfer the vegetable mixture to a dish and keep to one side.

Remove the lamb from the marinade and sauté in the casserole until browned all over. Spoon the marinade over the lamb. Cover with stock (bouillon) and add the bay leaves, salt and pepper and put back onto the heat. Stir in the vegetables and bring to the boil. Cover the casserole, transfer to the oven and cook for about 1½ hours until tender.

When the lamb is cooked, remove it from the pan. Skim off any fat with a big spoon, stir in the dissolved cornflour (cornstarch), bring to the boil and allow to bubble away until the sauce is reduced and thick but there is still enough to serve six.

Return the lamb to the casserole, spooning the sauce over the lamb, and reheat. Serve sprinkled with chopped parsley.

Pork Braised with Fennel and Artichoke Hearts

This light, Mediterranean-style casserole is ideal for summer lunches and is delicious served with steamed baby new potatoes and fresh summer peas. This dish freezes well but it can also be made 2 days in advance and kept in the refrigerator.

Serves 8

GF DF

4 tablespoons cold pressed extra virgin olive oil

1.2kg/2lb 10oz cubed pork, trimmed of fat

2 large fennel bulbs, trimmed and sliced

2 large onions, halved and sliced

2 garlic cloves, crushed

2 teaspoons ground coriander

Sea salt and freshly ground black pepper

Grated zest and juice of 2 unwaxed lemons

2 heaped tablespoons wheat-free flour mix*

250ml/1 cup dry white wine

250ml/1 cup allergy-free vegetable or chicken stock (bouillon)

2 x 400g/14oz cans artichoke hearts, drained

About 24 pitted black olives, in oil not vinegar

About 24 pitted green olives, in oil not vinegar

2 heaped tablespoons chopped fresh parsley

2 heaped tablespoons chopped fresh coriander (cilantro) leaves

---

* coeliacs please use gluten-free ingredients

Preheat the oven to 180°C/350°F/Gas mark 4.

Heat half the oil in an oven- and flame-proof casserole, add the pork and brown all over. Transfer the meat to a plate and sauté the fennel and onion in the oil until softened but not browned. Add the garlic, coriander, salt and pepper and cook for a few minutes. Stir in the lemon zest, return the pork to the casserole, sprinkle with the flour and stir. Cook for a couple of minutes before stirring in the wine, stock (bouillon) and half the lemon juice.

Bring the casserole to the boil, cover and transfer it to the oven to cook for about 1½ hours until the meat is tender. Remove the casserole from the oven and stir in the artichoke hearts, olives, remaining lemon juice and parsley and leave the casserole for about 10 minutes. Serve sprinkled with coriander (cilantro) leaves or cool and freeze.

If you want to keep the casserole for 2 days simply let it cool and refrigerate until 1 hour before needed. At this point, stir in the final ingredients (artichokes, olives etc.) and reheat at the given temperature for about 40 minutes. Sprinkle with coriander (cilantro) leaves and serve.

Pheasant Casserole with Caramelized Walnuts

We usually take black peppercorns for granted in any recipe but in this one they play a very important part. You can make the same peppery dish with guinea fowl.

Serves 6

GF   DF

2 heaped tablespoons wheat-free flour mix*

Sea salt and freshly ground black pepper

3 small pheasants, halved or very plump ones jointed into 6 breasts and 6 legs

3 tablespoons cold pressed extra virgin olive oil

115g/4oz finely chopped bacon or lardons

1 large onion, finely chopped

115g/1 cup shelled walnuts

Plenty of coarsely crushed black peppercorns

55g/⅓ cup unrefined golden granulated sugar

30g/1oz organic butter or dairy-free margarine

250ml/1 cup sherry

500ml/2 cups allergy-free pheasant or chicken stock

2 heaped tablespoons chopped fresh parsley

Optional

1 heaped tablespoon pure cornflour (cornstarch) dissolved in a little cold filtered water

*** coeliacs please use gluten-free ingredients**

Preheat the oven to 180°C/350°F/Gas mark 4.

Mix the flour with salt and pepper on a plate and dust the pheasant portions in the mixture.

Heat half the oil in a non-stick frying pan (skillet), add the bacon bits and fry until crispy. Transfer to a heatproof casserole using a slotted spoon and keep to one side. Reduce the heat under the pan, add the onion and cook until lightly golden but not browned. Add the onion to the plate of bacon bits. Heat the remaining oil in the pan, add the pheasant portions and brown on all sides. Add to the onions and bacon bits. Lastly, sauté the walnuts with the black peppercorns, sugar and butter or margarine until caramelized and golden brown. Add the nuts to the casserole.

Pour the sherry into the pan and shake over the heat, scraping in all the bits for a minute or two and then pour the juices into the casserole. Pour the pheasant or chicken stock (bouillon) over the pheasant mixture and mix all the ingredients together using a wooden spoon.

Cover the casserole with a lid, cook for about 55 minutes until the pheasants are tender and you have a delicious thick and glossy sauce. If the sauce is not thick then simply thicken it immediately it comes out of the oven with the dissolved cornflour (cornstarch). Serve sprinkled with parsley.

Summer Mexican Beef Wraps

Wraps are all the rage and make a great change from sandwiches for lunch but for coeliacs and those with a wheat intolerance they're another forbidden temptation. Now, however, you can make your own.
Vegetarians can make these with guacamole and roast sweet peppers (bell peppers) instead of beef.

Serves 4 (2 wraps each) (double the ingredients for picnic menu page 296 however, children only need one each)

GF   DF

Wraps

200g/2 cups wheat-free flour mix*
2 teaspoons wheat-free baking powder*
2 large organic free-range eggs
400ml/1½ cups organic milk or organic unsweetened dairy-free soya milk
Sea salt and freshly ground black pepper
A little cold pressed extra virgin olive oil for frying the pancakes

Filling

A little chopped chilli in oil
Homemade mayonnaise or any brand of wheat-free mayonnaise*
1 romaine lettuce, shredded
Cherry vine tomatoes, quartered
2 small ripe avocados, cut into thin slices and tossed with the fresh juice of 1 lime
4 large thick slices leftover roast beef, trimmed of fat and cut into short strips or 2 cooked beef steaks of your choice, sliced into short strips

Optional

Crème fraîche or Tofutti Sour Supreme dairy-free sour cream alternative (see page 305 for stockist)
2 heaped tablespoons chopped fresh coriander (cilantro) leaves

* coeliacs please use gluten-free ingredients

Make the wraps first. Sift the flour and baking powder into a bowl. Make a well in the centre and break in the eggs. Gradually whisk in the milk to make a thick batter and season with salt and pepper. Heat the oil in a large frying pan (skillet), over medium heat, ladle about a tablespoon of the batter into the pan and swirl around until you have an even-sized pancake. Cook for a couple of minutes until you see bubbles appearing on the surface. Flip the pancake over using an oiled palette knife and cook for a few minutes until golden brown. Transfer the pancake onto a large sheet of non-stick baking parchment (wax paper) and continue to make the remaining seven.

Mix the chilli with the mayonnaise and some salt and pepper. Arrange a little lettuce, some of the mayonnaise, a few tomato quarters, some avocado slices and some strips of cold beef or warm steak over each pancake and fold the edges over into a wrap.

Eat straight away, served with a large dollop of crème fraîche or Sour Supreme and sprinkled with the chopped coriander (cilantro).

If you are keeping the wrap for a lunch box or for later in the day, secure the wrap by rolling it up in clingfilm (plastic wrap). Keep it chilled until needed. Eat on the day of making.

Pork Valdostana

This simple pork dish can be prepared earlier in the day and cooked at the last minute. Pork Valdostana is delicious served with sauté potatoes and grilled vine tomatoes.

Serves 4

GF Q&E

---

4 x 225g/8oz loin pork chops (if you buy them from a butcher, ask him to French trim the chops)
4 thin slices prosciutto
4 fresh sage leaves
4 thin slices organic fontina cheese
2 tablespoons organic rice flour
Sea salt and freshly ground black pepper
2 tablespoons cold pressed extra virgin olive oil
30g/1oz organic butter
4 tablespoons Marsala or sherry

Preheat the oven to 220°C/425°F/Gas mark 7.

To trim the chops yourself, you'll need a sharp knife. Use this to cut around the lower part of the bone, scraping off the fat and all the meat; then trim off the fat from the lean loin part of the chop. Flatten the meat with a few bashes of a meat mallet or rolling pin.

Place a slice of prosciutto on a clean surface and place one sage leaf and a slice of cheese on top. Place the meaty bit of the chop over the top and wrap the prosciutto around the chop. Mix the flour with salt and pepper on a flat plate, coat the wrapped chop in the seasoned flour and shake to remove excess flour.

Heat the oil and butter in a large ovenproof frying pan (skillet), add the chops and fry them on both sides for a couple of minutes until browned. Pour over the Marsala or sherry and bring to the boil. Transfer to the oven and bake for about 20 minutes until the chops are cooked through and tender.

Serve the chops with the juices spooned over.

Chicken Kiev in Parma Ham

This is a health-conscious version of an old favourite. You need to make the garlic butter at least 4 hours in advance or preferably the day before in order for it to be completely frozen.

Serves 4

GF **DF**

Garlic butter

110g/½ cup soft organic butter or dairy-free margarine
2 large garlic cloves, crushed
Sea salt and freshly ground black pepper
5 tablespoons finely chopped parsley leaves
2 tablespoons finely chopped basil leaves

Chicken

4 free-range organic chicken breasts, skin and fat removed
12 thin slices Parma ham
Olive oil for brushing
60g/2oz pack prepared wild rocket (arugula)
150g/5½oz pack sunblush tomatoes in oil, drained

Preheat the oven to 180°C/350°F/Gas mark 4.

Make the garlic butter or margarine by mashing all the ingredients together in a small bowl with a small wooden spoon or, alternatively, in a food processor for a few seconds. Shape the mixture with clean hands into 4 equal sausage shapes, then squash them down with your hands, so that they flatten slightly. Wrap each one in clingfilm (plastic wrap) and freeze until rock hard.

Using a sharp knife, slice the chicken breast down the length first, but not all the way through, and then deep into the width of the breast, but again not all the way through. Insert the frozen garlic margarine or butter into the pocket. Seal up the flesh, carefully enclosing the filling, and bind it all together by wrapping each breast up in 3 slices of Parma ham. Brush the ham with a little oil, place in an ovenproof dish and bake for 25 minutes in the centre of the oven.

As soon as the chicken breasts are ready, arrange the rocket (arugula) between 4 plates and divide the sunblush tomatoes between them. Place a chicken breast on each salad, spoon over all the juices and serve immediately.

Rack of Lamb with Courgettes, Broad Beans and Mint

Having spent 10 years living near the borders of Shropshire and Wales, I have been used to the delicious Welsh lamb that our farmers produce each spring. This recipe melts in the mouth but needs to be served pink to get the best results.

Serves 6

GF   DF   RF

2 racks organic lamb (6–7 bones in each one), for a less expensive recipe use a 1.5kg (3lb 5oz) leg of organic lamb

2 heaped teaspoons Dijon mustard*

1 heaped tablespoon fresh thyme leaves

125g/4½oz pancetta cubes or bacon cubes

455g/1lb courgettes (zucchini), cut into cubes

2 tablespoons cold pressed extra virgin olive oil

400g/14oz can artichoke hearts or bottoms, drained and quartered

200g/1 cup baby broad (fava) beans, blanched for 1 minute in boiling water, drained and rinsed under cold running water

1 large garlic clove, crushed

Sea salt and freshly ground black pepper

300ml/1⅓ cups allergy-free chicken or lamb stock (bouillon)

7g/¼oz mint leaves, chopped

* coeliacs please use gluten-free ingredients

Preheat the oven to 180°C/350°F/Gas mark 4.

Spread the mustard over the skin of the lamb. Sprinkle with thyme, salt and pepper, and place the racks of lamb, mustard side up, in a roasting pan. Roast in the oven for about 35 minutes, or until it is as pink as you like it, but don't forget that it will continue to cook for a few minutes once it is out of the oven. Remove it from the pan and leave it to rest for about 10 minutes. (If you are cooking the leg of lamb this will take about 45 minutes.)

While the lamb is cooking, fry the pancetta and courgettes (zucchini) in the oil in a non-stick frying pan (skillet) over a medium heat until dark brown at the edges. Add the artichokes, stir in the broad (fava) beans, garlic, and season to taste. Add the stock (bouillon) and simmer for 10 minutes. Mix in the mint leaves, add any juices from the lamb and keep the sauce warm.

Carve the rack of lamb and arrange 2 cutlets on a bed of the vegetable mixture on each plate. Serve immediately, accompanied by a big continental dressed salad. (Carve the leg of lamb, serve all the vegetable mixture on one large serving dish and arrange the slices of lamb along the length of it.)

Beef with Celeriac Mash and Tomato and Olive Compote

I made this dish for my husband's birthday recently and it was utterly gorgeous, not only was the meat organic but properly hung and full of flavour. We eat far less meat than we used to but when we do, we really go for it!

GF **DF**

Serves 6

Meat and marinade

1kg/2¼lb trimmed organic beef fillet steak, or sirloin steak

1 tablespoon finely chopped fresh rosemary leaves

2 garlic cloves, crushed

60ml/¼ cup cold pressed extra virgin olive oil

Sea salt and freshly ground black pepper

Tomato and olive compote

1 red onion, finely chopped

2 tablespoons cold pressed extra virgin olive oil

8 large peeled plum tomatoes, with the tops removed, cut into quarters, seeds and pith removed

1 garlic clove, crushed

1 teaspoon fresh thyme leaves

125ml/½ cup allergy-free vegetable stock (bouillon) or water

1 tablespoon balsamic vinegar

85g/¾ cup pitted black olives*, rinsed under cold water and then halved

24 basil leaves, torn

Celeriac mash

I celeriac, peeled and cut into cubes
Juice of ½ a lemon
30g/2 tablespoons organic butter or dairy-free margarine
Grated nutmeg
Cayenne pepper
I heaped teaspoon fresh thyme leaves
20g/¾oz parsley, finely chopped for decoration

coeliacs please use gluten-free ingredients

Preheat the oven to 200°C/400°F/Gas mark 6.

Marinate the meat the night before cooking. Mix the rosemary, garlic, olive oil and seasoning in a little bowl. Lay the steak in a roasting pan and spread the marinade evenly all over it. Keep the steak covered and chilled in the refrigerator.

Make the compote. Gently cook the onions in the oil in a non-stick frying pan (skillet) over medium heat for about 10 minutes, until softened but not brown. Add the tomatoes, garlic, thyme, vegetable stock (bouillon), salt, pepper and balsamic vinegar and cook over a medium heat for a further 30 minutes, stirring from time to time. Add the olives and basil, cover the pan with a lid and leave until needed.

Meanwhile, cook the celeriac in a saucepan of boiling water with the lemon juice until soft. Drain and mash until smooth. Beat in the margarine, salt, pepper, nutmeg, cayenne and thyme. Keep warm until needed.

Roast the fillet steak in the marinade in the oven for about 15 minutes for blue, 20 minutes for very pink, or 25 minutes for pink (add about 5 minutes more cooking if using sirloin). Remove the steak from the oven and let it sit for 5 minutes before carving, as it will continue to cook at this stage.

Place a couple of large spoonfuls of the mash on to the centre of each warm plate. Carve the fillet, allowing 2 thin slices for each person and arrange them across the mash. Spoon a dollop of compote beside it and sprinkle with some parsley. Serve immediately with a bowl of dressed green salad leaves, for example rocket (arugula), baby spinach and watercress.

Duck Breasts with Marmalade and Mango

Orange and duck has been an unfailing combination for a very long time, used by the greatest and the most famous of chefs and cooks. This is my simplified and updated version, which is very quick and easy.

Serves 2

GF   DF   Q&E

Sprinkling of ground allspice

2 duck breasts, washed then dried with absorbent kitchen paper

Sea salt and freshly ground black pepper

½ ripe, medium-sized mango, peeled and flesh chopped into small cubes

1 heaped tablespoon pale orange marmalade

Juice of ½ a large orange

Juice of ½ a small lemon

Lightly sprinkle the allspice all over the duck breasts and then gently rub it in with clean fingers. Season with salt and pepper. Fry the duck, skin down, in a non-stick frying pan (skillet) over a high heat for 6 minutes. Watch that it does not burn and turn the heat down a fraction if necessary. It should be dark and crispy. Meanwhile, mix the mango, marmalade and orange juice together in a bowl with a little salt and plenty of black pepper.

Drain the fat out of the pan and discard it. Turn the breasts over and pour in the mango mixture, reduce the heat to medium and cook for 5 minutes. Lift out the duck breasts and let them sit on a carving board for 1 minute. Meanwhile, stir the lemon juice into the sauce.

Carve the breasts into a fan shape with a very sharp knife. Lift each carved breast onto a warm plate and spoon the hot sauce around the base and one side. Serve immediately with steamed green vegetables.

Chicken and Basil Curry

Green curry paste is available in all good supermarkets or oriental stores and gives a lovely mellow flavour and silky texture. You can make a delicious vegetarian version of this recipe using green beans, broad (fava) beans and courgettes (zucchini) instead of the chicken.

GF   DF   RF

Serves 6

1 tablespoon green curry paste*

2 tablespoons cold pressed extra virgin olive oil

2 large garlic cloves, crushed

2 stems lemon grass, finely sliced

2 lime leaves, shredded

2 x 400ml/14fl oz cans half-fat coconut milk (Blue Dragon)

15g/½oz fresh basil leaves, coarsely shredded

6 large organic chicken breasts, cut into diagonal pieces or 1 supermarket ready-cooked chicken, skin removed and carved into 6 pieces

2 green mild chillies, seeded and finely chopped

2 tablespoons Thai fish sauce*

Finely grated rind and juice of 1 unwaxed lime

15g/½oz fresh coriander (cilantro) leaves, chopped

* coeliacs please use gluten-free ingredients

Fry the curry paste in the oil in a big non-stick frying pan (skillet) over a medium heat for about 2 minutes, stirring occasionally. Add the garlic, lemon grass, lime leaves and half the coconut milk to the paste and cook for about 5 minutes. Stir in the basil, chicken, chilli and remaining coconut milk. Simmer for about 20 minutes, by which time the smaller raw pieces will be cooked and the larger cooked chicken pieces heated through. Remove from the heat, stir in the Nam Pla (fish sauce) and the grated rind and juice of the lime.

As this curry is almost soup-like, it is a good idea to serve it in warm bowls and then sprinkle with the chopped coriander (cilantro). If you are serving steamed fragrant Thai rice, then the rice will soak up the curry sauce and warm plates will be fine for serving.

Chicken with Rosemary and Verjuice

We are used to the concentrated and deep flavour of balsamic vinegar, the lighter sherry vinegar and oriental rice vinegar, but now we are about to join the verjuice (vert jus) craze.

In French this literally means the 'green juice', which is extracted from unripe grapes. Ever since the Romans introduced vines to England, this juice has been used for cooking, and this only stopped when the vineyards went into decline. Once again, we have a thriving winemaking industry and our vineyards can produce this culinary delight to use in recipes from all over the world.

Serves 4

GF   DF   RF

60g/generous ⅓ cup raisins

200ml/¾ cup verjuice (available from Sainsbury's special selection)

2 teaspoons finely chopped rosemary

I large garlic clove, crushed

Sea salt and freshly ground black pepper

4 organic chicken breasts, skin and fat removed

I tablespoon cold pressed extra virgin olive oil

60g/generous ⅓ cup pine nuts

I tablespoon finely chopped parsley

Soak the raisins in the verjuice in a bowl overnight. The next day, stir in the rosemary, garlic, salt and pepper.

Arrange the chicken breasts in a shallow dish that is just big enough to prevent the breasts from touching each other. Pour the verjuice mixture over the chicken and leave to marinate for the rest of the day. Keep covered and chilled in the refrigerator.

In a non-stick frying pan (skillet), sauté the chicken breasts in the oil for 5 minutes on each side over a medium heat. Add the pine nuts, cook for a couple of minutes, then add the verjuice mixture.

Simmer for about 10 minutes until the chicken breasts are completely cooked. Lift the chicken from the pan on to warm plates. Spoon the sauce over the chicken, sprinkle with parsley and serve immediately with a selection of vegetables.

Salads ...

Caramelized Salmon and Lime Salad

Salmon works very well with Thai-style ingredients in this easy and quick dish.

Serves 4

GF   DF   RF   Q&E

Salad

255g/9oz packet bean sprouts
15g/½oz fresh mint leaves, finely chopped
15g/½oz fresh coriander (cilantro) leaves, finely chopped
1 teaspoon cold pressed extra virgin olive oil
4 thick salmon fillets, skin and bones removed
1 unwaxed lime, cut into quarters

Sauce

1 mild red chilli, finely chopped
5cm/2in piece fresh root ginger, thickly grated (use less for a milder taste)
1½ tablespoons runny honey
1 garlic clove, crushed
4 spring onions (scallions), trimmed and finely sliced
1 tablespoon Thai fish sauce*
Finely grated rind and 1 tablespoon juice from an unwaxed lime
1 tablespoon soy sauce*
Sea salt and freshly ground black pepper

* coeliacs please use gluten-free ingredients

Mix the bean sprouts with the mint and coriander (cilantro) leaves and arrange on four plates. Place all the sauce ingredients in a small pan and warm through.

Meanwhile, heat the oil in a non-stick frying pan (skillet) and, over medium-high heat, cook the salmon so that it is golden brown on the outside but only just cooked through inside.

Arrange the salmon at a jaunty angle over the salad and spoon over the sauce. Serve immediately with the lime quarters.

Piedmontese Peppers

You can roast the peppers one day in advance, cool, cover and chill them. The smooth sweetness of the peppers contrasts well with the crumbly sharpness of the feta cheese. Even the dairy-free version gives a good contrast of textures and flavours.

GF   DF

Serves 6 as an appetizer or side salad

---

3 large red peppers (bell peppers), halved and seeded

55g/2oz can anchovies in oil, drained

1 garlic clove, crushed

200g/7oz vine cherry tomatoes, quartered

2 tablespoons cold pressed extra virgin olive oil

1 tablespoon balsamic vinegar

Freshly ground black pepper

200g/7oz packet organic feta cheese, crumbled into bite-size pieces or 150g/5oz jar Redwood dairy-free feta cheese in oil (see page 305 for stockist)

6 small handfuls fresh baby spinach leaves

12 fresh basil leaves

Preheat the oven to 200°C/400°F/Gas mark 6.

Put the peppers, skin side down on a baking tray. Cut the anchovies into 24 strips – you can cut the big ones into three and the smaller ones in half.

In a bowl, mix the garlic, tomatoes, oil and vinegar and season with pepper. Spoon a little of the mixture into the cavity of each pepper. Decorate with four strips of anchovy in a crisscross pattern, add the crumbled cheese and bake for about 30 minutes until the peppers are tender.

Arrange the spinach leaves on a large serving dish. Place the peppers on top, sprinkle over all the cooking juices from the peppers and then decorate with the basil leaves.

For a delicious lunch for three people, serve with warm wheat- or gluten-free bread and a salad.

Caesar Salad with Parmesan Crisps

The Parmesan crisps are quick and easy to make and you can serve them with any sort of salad combination, such as avocado and pine nuts or olives and roasted peppers.

Serves 6

GF   Q&E

Crisps
55g/2oz piece Parmesan cheese, finely grated

Dressing
2 organic free-range eggs, boiled for 2 minutes and cooled under cold running water

55g/2oz can anchovy fillets, drained and coarsely chopped

1 garlic clove, peeled

4 tablespoons cold pressed extra virgin olive oil

Finely grated rind and juice of 1 unwaxed lemon

1 teaspoon unrefined golden caster (superfine) sugar

A generous dash of Worcestershire sauce*

Freshly ground black pepper

2 heaped tablespoons crème fraîche or a light mayonnaise*

2 heaped tablespoons finely grated fresh Parmesan

Salad
3 very thick slices of wheat-free white bread*, crusts removed (see page 304 for stockist)

3–4 tablespoons cold pressed extra virgin olive oil

2 large romaine lettuces, sliced into bite-size pieces

* coeliacs please use gluten-free ingredients

Preheat the oven to 200°C/400°F/Gas mark 6.

First make the crisps. Line two baking sheets with non-stick baking parchment (wax paper) or Bake-O-Glide. Spoon the Parmesan onto the baking sheets in six 8cm/3in rounds, leaving room for them to spread during cooking. Bake them for about 5 minutes until golden.

Cool the crisps for 30 seconds then, using a palette knife, lift each one onto a wire rack. Leave them to cool completely before lifting off the rack.

Now make the dressing for the salad. Carefully peel the eggs, place in a food processor or blender with all the remaining dressing ingredients and process until smooth and well blended. Set aside.

Cut the bread for the salad into very small croûtons, heat the oil and fry the croûtons until they are golden on all sides. Drain the croûtons on absorbent kitchen paper, place in a bowl with the salad leaves and toss with the dressing.

Divide the Caesar salad mixture between the plates and serve with a Parmesan crisp jauntily balanced on top.

Please note that this recipe contains lightly cooked egg.

Chicken, Broad Bean and Bacon Salad

You can choose all sorts of seasonal salad leaves, such a dandelion or rocket (arugula), for this lovely summer salad. I love sitting on our veranda, looking at the view and shelling broad (fava) beans into a bowl whilst chatting to friends and enjoying a glass or two of chilled white wine.

Serves 4 (double the recipe for the menu on page 296)

GF · DF · Q&E

---

4 x 170g/6oz boned and skinless chicken breasts

Sea salt and freshly ground black pepper

3 tablespoons cold pressed extra virgin olive oil, plus extra for brushing

115g/4oz smoked rindless back bacon

340g/2 cups baby broad (fava) beans, fresh or frozen

2 tablespoons red wine vinegar

1 tablespoon chopped chives

4 handfuls ready-prepared salad leaves

Season the chicken breasts with a little salt and pepper and brush with a little oil. Cook the chicken under a hot grill (broiler) or on a hot barbecue. When the chicken breasts are browned on one side, turn them over and add the pieces of bacon to the grill (broiler) pan and cook until crispy on both sides. Snip the cooked bacon into small pieces and leave to one side. When the chicken breasts are cooked through, keep them warm.

Cook the broad (fava) beans in boiling water for a few minutes until tender, drain and refresh under cold running water. Meanwhile, mix the wine vinegar with the 3 tablespoons of oil, some salt and pepper, the chives, bacon bits and the warm beans in a bowl.

To serve, place a handful of salad on each plate, sprinkle with the bean and bacon dressing and place a chicken breast at a jaunty angle on top of the salad.

Warm Bread, Bacon and Poached Egg Salad

Here is a wonderfully French way of enjoying bacon and eggs – it's slightly healthier than the conventional British method of serving bacon and eggs, as they are cooked in olive oil and served on a bed of fresh salad.

Serves 2

GF   DF   Q&E

---

2 slices very thick white gluten-free bread, crusts removed and discarded (see page 304 for stockist)

4 tablespoons cold pressed extra virgin olive oil

4 thick slices rindless back bacon, very thinly sliced or diced

2 extra large organic free-range eggs

1 small garlic clove, crushed

2 tablespoons balsamic vinegar

Sea salt and freshly ground black pepper

1 heart of romaine lettuce, trimmed and sliced

Bring a small pan of water to the boil. Meanwhile, chop the bread into bite-size pieces to make the croûtons. Fry them in half the oil in a large non-stick frying pan (skillet), over moderate heat, until they are golden and crispy. Transfer the croûtons to a plate and fry the bacon in the same pan.

Meanwhile, poach the eggs in the boiling water for a few minutes – or however you like them cooked. Stir the garlic into the bacon and cook for a minute before adding the vinegar, salt and pepper and the remaining olive oil. Shake vigorously and remove from the heat.

Arrange the lettuce on each plate, sprinkle with the croûtons, the bacon and dressing and top with a poached egg. Serve immediately.

Chickpea, Avocado and Sweet Pepper Salad

Salads can sometimes leave me feeling rather hungry but the chickpeas (garbanzos) in this salad always fill me up. I usually serve this salad with the Rye and Barley Soda Bread* on page 271 or the Olive and Rosemary Bread* on page 274.

GF   **DF**   **V**   **Q&E**

Serves 2 as a main course or 4 as an appetizer

4 handfuls baby spinach leaves

400g/14oz can chickpeas (garbanzos), drained and rinsed under cold running water

½ x 375g/13oz jar baby sweet mild spicy peppers (Peppadew)* (check other brands are not pickled in malt vinegar), drained and coarsely chopped or halve, roast, skin and seed one red and one yellow sweet pepper (bell pepper), and coarsely chop

1 small garlic clove for 2 people or 1 large for 4 people, crushed

Finely grated rind of ½ an unwaxed lemon

As much finely chopped chilli as you fancy

2 tablespoons cold pressed extra virgin olive oil

2 heaped tablespoons chopped coriander (cilantro) leaves

1 small ripe avocado for 2 people or 1 large one for 4 people, flesh coarsely chopped

Sea salt and freshly ground black pepper

* coeliacs please use gluten-free ingredients

Arrange a handful of spinach leaves on each plate. In a bowl, mix the chickpeas (garbanzos), sweet peppers, garlic, grated lemon rind and juice, chilli, oil, coriander (cilantro) and avocado. Season to taste with salt and pepper and spoon the mixture onto each pile of spinach leaves. Serve with wheat- or gluten-free warm bread.

Puy Lentil Salad

Pumpkin seed oil is a new discovery for me; it is very dark and syrupy but excellent with strong-tasting salads and firmer textures. It can be drizzled over any pulses, roasted vegetables or, of course, over baked pumpkin or squashes.

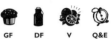

Serves 4–6

GF   DF   V   Q&E

2 x 300g/10½oz cans Puy lentils, drained and rinsed under cold running water
1 garlic clove, crushed
2 tablespoons cider or white wine vinegar
3 tablespoons pumpkin oil
½ small red onion, finely diced
100g/3½oz carton sunblush tomatoes (semi-dried tomatoes in flavoured oil or vacuum packed), halved
Sea salt and freshly ground black pepper
2 heaped tablespoons pumpkin seeds
2 heaped tablespoons chopped fresh parsley

Mix the lentils and garlic together in a salad bowl. Stir in the vinegar, oil, onion and tomatoes and season to taste with salt and pepper. Sprinkle with pumpkin seeds and parsley and serve with fresh, warm wheat- or gluten-free bread.

Roasted Vegetable and Goats' Cheese Salad

Mediterranean vegetables taste sweet and mellow when roasted with olive oil and a little seasoning. You can experiment with different goat or sheep cheeses and use different herbs.

Serves 4 (double the recipe for the menu on page 296)

GF   V   Q&E

---

2 large courgettes (zucchini), trimmed and cut into fairly large wedges

1 large or 3 very small fennel bulbs, trimmed and cut into fairly large wedges

1 sweet red pepper (bell pepper), seeded and cut into quarters

1 sweet yellow pepper (bell pepper), seeded and cut into quarters

1 medium red onion, quartered

6 tablespoons cold pressed extra virgin olive oil

2 garlic cloves, finely sliced

Sea salt and freshly ground black pepper

4 thick slices of round, firm goats' cheese

Juice of ½ a lemon

Fresh basil leaves, shredded

Preheat the oven to 220°C/425°F/Gas mark 7.

Place all the vegetables in a large non-stick roasting tin (pan) with the oil, garlic and plenty of salt and pepper and roast them for about 25 minutes until soft and tinged with golden brown. Turn all the vegetables over and roast for another 20 minutes. Place four slices of cheese on top of the vegetables, making sure that they are far enough apart so that you can easily transfer the cheese and vegetables onto four warm serving plates.

Roast the cheese and vegetables for about 5 minutes until the cheese is just melted and quickly transfer onto the plates. Serve sprinkled with a little lemon juice and the basil leaves.

Green and Yellow Wax Bean Salad

This is a jazzy combination of beans – if you can't find the yellow beans, just use any type of fine green beans. Serve this salad with fresh warm bread to mop up the dressing.

Serves 6

GF   DF   V   Q&E

225g/8oz green beans, washed, topped and tailed
225g/8oz yellow wax beans, washed, topped and tailed
1 tablespoon balsamic vinegar
3 tablespoons walnut oil
½ red onion, finely chopped
Sea salt and freshly ground black pepper
55g/scant 1½ cup chopped walnuts
2 heaped tablespoons chopped fresh parsley

Cook the beans in two separate pans of boiling water until both sets of beans are al dente. Drain the beans and refresh under cold running water. Make the dressing by whisking the vinegar with the oil, onion, seasoning, walnuts and parsley until you have a glossy sauce. Toss the beans and the dressing together in a serving bowl, cover and chill until needed. Serve at room temperature.

Summer Pilaf with Hummus Dressing

This is a healthy quick-fix lunch and is delicious served with warm, homemade wheat-free bread.

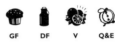

Serves 2

100g/½ cup brown basmati rice

1 medium courgette (zucchini), finely chopped

1 tablespoon cold pressed extra virgin olive oil

115g/1 cup cooked peas or baby broad (fava) beans

Sea salt and freshly ground black pepper

155g/1 cup cooked chickpeas (garbanzos)

30g/⅓ cup chopped walnut pieces

¼ small cucumber, peeled and finely chopped

Juice of 1 lemon

2 tablespoons cold pressed extra virgin olive oil or avocado oil

2 heaped tablespoons ready-made hummus*

1 tablespoon chopped fresh coriander (cilantro) leaves

---

* coeliacs please use gluten-free ingredients

Cook the rice in boiling water until soft, then drain and refresh under cold running water. Meanwhile, fry the courgettes (zucchini) in the tablespoon of oil until soft, golden and crispy. Cook the peas or broad (fava) beans until tender in boiling water, then drain and refresh under cold running water. Mix all the cooked vegetables together in a salad bowl.

Season the vegetables with salt and pepper and mix in the chickpeas (garbanzos), walnuts and cucumber. In a small bowl, whisk together the lemon juice, oil, hummus and coriander (cilantro) until combined.

Divide the salad between two plates, pour the dressing over the salads and serve.

Spinach, Mushroom and Garlic Croûton Salad

This is a quick and easy salad that is ideal served before spicy food or fish dishes. Any leftovers can be taken to work the next day.

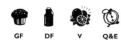

Serves 6

GF   DF   V   Q&E

130g/4½oz gluten-free white bread with crusts removed (see page 304 for stockist)

2 large garlic cloves, crushed

Plenty of cold pressed extra virgin olive oil

455g/1lb baby mushrooms, wiped clean and sliced

Sea salt and freshly ground black pepper

100g/3½oz packet semi-dried tomatoes

Balsamic vinegar

115g/4oz packet prepared baby spinach leaves

Cut the bread into bite-size cubes. Heat the oil in a non-stick frying pan (skillet), add the cubes of bread and crushed garlic and fry until the bread is golden brown all over. Drain the croûtons on kitchen paper. Add the mushrooms to the same pan and fry until tinged with gold, adding more oil as needed. Season with salt and pepper, stir in the tomatoes and drizzle with balsamic vinegar according to taste. Cook for a few minutes.

Arrange the spinach leaves on plates. Sprinkle with the mushrooms, tomatoes, juices and croûtons and serve immediately, drizzled with extra oil and black pepper if needed.

Asparagus Salad with Coriander and Ginger Dressing

This salad is made up of a delicious combination of vegetables, but you can always make another kind of salad – for example, a prawn (shrimp) or chicken and avocado salad – and just use the delicious dressing from this recipe.

GF	DF	V	RF	Q&E

Serves 4

2 large red onions, cut into 10
Cold pressed extra virgin olive oil
1 teaspoon fresh thyme leaves
200g/7oz pack prepared fresh asparagus tips
3 medium courgettes (zucchini)

Dressing
Juice of 1 lemon
1 teaspoon Dijon mustard*
1 tablespoon clear honey
4 tablespoons bottled fat-free French dressing or cold pressed extra virgin olive oil
1 teaspoon coriander seeds
2 teaspoons finely grated root ginger
Sea salt and freshly ground black pepper
20g/¾oz chopped fresh parsley

coeliacs please use gluten-free ingredients

Preheat the oven to 200°C/400°F/Gas mark 6.

Put the onions in a baking tray, drizzle with oil and sprinkle with thyme. Bake them for 20–30 minutes until blackened at the edges but soft in the centre. Meanwhile, cook the asparagus in boiling water until just tender. Drain and refresh them under cold running water.

    Cut each courgette (zucchini) into about 10 diagonal chunks and cook in a pan of boiling water until just cooked through but still slightly crunchy. Drain and refresh under cold running water. Arrange the hot onions and both the vegetables on a serving dish. Now make the dressing by whisking all the ingredients together (except the parsley) in a bowl in the given order. Pour the dressing all over the salad, sprinkle with parsley and serve or cover and chill until needed.

Artichoke, Butter Bean and Fennel Salad

Although they have the flavour of globe artichokes, Jerusalem artichokes are, in fact, a relative of the sunflower. Jerusalem artichokes appear in November and then throughout the winter. These artichokes are warming and comforting, whereas artichoke hearts are light and flowery, and so are ideal for the summer months.

Serves 4

GF · DF · V · RF · Q&E

2 red onions, cut into 6
Plenty of cold pressed extra virgin olive oil
Sea salt and freshly ground black pepper
A sprinkling of herbes de Provence (mixed herbs can be used as an alternative)
455g/1lb Jerusalem artichokes, peeled or 400g/14oz can artichoke hearts, or bottoms, drained, rinsed under cold water and halved
2 courgettes (zucchini), thickly sliced
400g/14oz can butter (lima) beans, drained and rinsed under cold water
60g/2oz prepared wild rocket (arugula)
1 large fennel bulb, outer layers removed, then trimmed and thinly sliced
15g/½oz fresh basil leaves, shredded
Finely grated rind and juice of 1 unwaxed lemon

Preheat the oven to 200°C/400°F/Gas mark 6.

Roast the onions in a baking tray with a drizzle of oil, a sprinkling of salt and pepper and herbes de Provence until they are dark brown at the edges and soft in the centre.

Put a pan of water on to boil. Drop the Jerusalem artichokes into the water and simmer for about 15 minutes, depending on their size. Drain and leave to cool.

Meanwhile, cook the courgette (zucchini) in another pan of boiling water until al dente, then allow to cool.

Mix the butter (lima) beans and rocket (arugula) with the fennel and basil leaves in a big salad bowl. Add the artichoke hearts if you are using them, or the cooled Jerusalem artichokes and the red onions and courgettes (zucchini). Season to taste with salt and freshly ground black pepper, the grated rind and lemon juice and some oil.

Toss the salad and serve straightaway. For a main course, serve with a baked potato or a potato salad.

Super Summer Mixed Salad

Ensure you use fresh and crisp ingredients for the salad as these provide the maximum nutrients as well as the best flavours and textures.

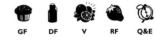

GF   DF   V   RF   Q&E

Serves 1

Salad

80g/½ cup grated raw beetroot (beet)

40g/⅓ cup finely sliced radishes

30g/½ cup finely sliced celery

40g/½ cup finely shredded cabbage leaves

20g/¾oz trimmed watercress

60g/1 cup sprouts – use any kind or combination: alfalfa, bean sprouts, mung, chickpeas (garbanzos), lentils

40g/½ cup grated carrots

1 thinly sliced vine tomato

50g/⅓ cup thinly sliced cucumber

Dressing

Dash of cold pressed extra virgin olive oil

A little fresh lemon or lime juice

½ small garlic clove, crushed (optional and according to taste)

Little minced chilli in oil or freshly chopped chilli (optional and according to taste)

Sea salt and freshly ground black pepper

Combine all the prepared salad ingredients in a bowl. Toss in the oil and lemon or lime juice according to preference, then toss in the garlic and chilli if you are using them. Season according to taste and serve immediately for ultimate freshness.

Vegetable Kebabs with Walnut and Rice Salad

There is absolutely no reason why kebabs should contain meat, so here are some which will be ideal if you have vegetarian guests or just want a lower fat and more easily digestible feast. You can cook the rice a day in advance and keep it covered and chilled until needed.

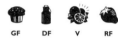

Serves 4

GF   DF   V   RF

2 heaped teaspoons fresh thyme leaves

1 large garlic clove, crushed

Light sprinkling dried chilli flakes, or minced chillies in oil

4 tablespoons cold pressed extra virgin olive oil

Sea salt and freshly ground black pepper

2 cobs sweetcorn, each cut into 4

1 courgette (zucchini), cut into 8

3 large flat mushrooms, peeled and stalk removed

1 green and 1 red pepper (bell pepper), seeded and cut into squares

8 fresh bay leaves

2 small red onions, cut into 8

Yogurt dip

400ml/1¾ cups virtually fat-free set natural (plain) sheep, goat or soy yogurt

1 small garlic clove, crushed

7g/¼oz chopped fresh mint leaves

7g/¼oz chopped fresh flat-leaf parsley leaves

Rice salad

170g/1 cup wild rice, cooked until tender then drained

170g/1 cup brown rice, cooked until tender then drained

60g/½ cup chopped walnuts

60g/½ cup halved almonds

60g/⅔ cup plump raisins

3 spring onions (scallions), chopped

7g/¼oz each chopped mint, chives and parsley

Grated rind and juice of 1 unwaxed orange

2 tablespoons cold pressed extra virgin olive oil

Minced chilli in oil

8 bamboo skewers, soaked in water for 5 minutes

First prepare the vegetable kebabs. Mix the thyme, garlic and chillies in a bowl with the olive oil and seasoning, and reserve. Cook the sweetcorn in boiling water for 10 minutes. Lift them out and leave to drain. Blanch the courgette (zucchini) in boiling water for 3 minutes. Drain, refresh under cold running water and set aside.

Blanch the mushrooms in boiling water for 1 minute. Drain, refresh under cold running water and set aside. When they are cool enough to touch, cut into quarters. Thread all the vegetables and a bay leaf on to each of the skewers. Brush with the garlic oil and cook for 10 minutes under a very hot grill (broiler). Turn them over, brush with the remaining sauce and cook for a further 10 minutes, or until the onions and peppers (bell peppers) are cooked through.

While the vegetables are cooking, make the yogurt dip. Combine all the ingredients in a bowl and season according to taste with salt and pepper. Alternatively, make this in advance and cover and chill until needed.

Quickly put the rice salad together by combining all the ingredients in the given order in a bowl and season to taste with salt and pepper. Transfer the rice salad on to a large serving dish. Arrange the cooked kebabs over the rice and serve immediately accompanied by the dip.

Chicken Liver and Cranberry Terrine with Broccoli and Almond Salad

One of my favourite activities in France is, I am sure you will not be surprised to hear, eating in restaurants. At lunchtime, I browse through the menu and hum and ha over the delicious choices, but often succumb to the most traditional terrine, which I know will always be perfect. This is my current favourite. It freezes well, so I make it all the time.

Serves 10

GF **DF**

Terrine

300g/10½oz rindless, smoked streaky bacon rashers (slices)

400g/14oz chicken livers, rinsed under cold running water and drained

500g/1lb 2oz extra-lean minced (ground) pork

1 onion, finely chopped

2 extra large garlic cloves, crushed

2 tablespoons chopped fresh parsley

1 tablespoon fresh thyme leaves or 1 teaspoon dried thyme

2 tablespoons brandy

75g/⅔ cup dried cranberries or 110g/4oz fresh or frozen cranberries, defrosted

Sea salt and freshly ground black pepper

3 bay leaves

Broccoli and almond salad

565g/1¼lbs prepared broccoli florets

285g/10oz mini vine tomatoes, halved

1 fennel bulb, trimmed, all tough layers removed and then finely sliced

About ½ a bottle of virtually fat-free French dressing (as much as you need to toss the salad) or cold pressed extra virgin olive oil

110g/¾ cup whole almonds with their skins, halved

15g/½oz chopped fresh flat-leaf parsley

1kg/2lb loaf tin (pan)

Preheat the oven to 180°C/350°F/Gas mark 4.

First make the terrine. Stretch most of the bacon across the base and up the sides of the loaf tin (pan), allowing the ends to hang over the edges. Place the remaining bacon in a food processor together with the livers, pork and onion, and chop finely but do not purée.

Turn the mixture into a bowl and mix in the garlic, herbs, brandy and cranberries and season with salt and pepper. Spoon the mixture into the prepared loaf tin (pan). Smooth the top of the mixture to the edges, lay the bay leaves on top and fold in the ends of the bacon. Cover with foil and stand in a roasting pan that is two-thirds filled with cold water. Cook in the oven for 2 hours, until the juices run clear when the middle of the loaf is pierced with a skewer. Remove the foil and cover with greaseproof (waxed) paper. Cover with a treble layer of foil, put a weight on top and leave it to cool, standing on a tray in case any juices escape. It should then be left to chill overnight.

Now make the broccoli and almond salad. Cook the broccoli in a pan of boiling water for 3 minutes, drain and refresh under cold running water. Transfer to a salad bowl, mix in the tomatoes and fennel, and sprinkle liberally with the dressing, almonds, salt, pepper and parsley.

Turn the terrine out on to a serving plate; serve with the broccoli and almond salad. A big green salad – spinach, rocket (arugula), chicory, salad leaves, cucumber and other favourites – lightly tossed in cold pressed extra virgin olive oil and black pepper is also a delicious accompaniment.

Sesame Salmon Fingers with Sugar Snap Salad

The good thing about salmon is that it is so filling, whether it is served hot or cold. I often make this dish for dinner for two and then invite a friend to lunch the next day, serving what is left as a delicious cold dish.

Serves 4

GF   DF   Q&E

Salad

255g/9oz dwarf green beans, top and tailed

350g/12oz fresh asparagus, cut into 15cm/6in lengths

200g/7oz prepared sugar snap peas

225g/8oz pack sunblush tomatoes in olive oil, coarsely chopped

2 tablespoons lemon juice

15g/½oz chives, chopped

Fish fingers

455g (1lb) salmon fillet, skinned and cut into 4 equal strips to look like thick fingers

2 heaped tablespoons wheat-free flour mix* spread over a dinner plate, seasoned with sea salt and freshly ground black pepper

2 large organic free-range eggs, beaten in a wide bowl

About 110g/4oz sesame seeds, more or less as you want, spread over a dinner plate

2 tablespoons cold pressed extra virgin olive oil

1 unwaxed lemon and 1 unwaxed lime, quartered for decoration and serving

* coeliacs please use gluten-free ingredients

The Big Book of Wheat-Free Cooking

First make the salad. Bring a big pan of water to the boil, add the beans and asparagus, and cook for 3 minutes. Then add the sugar snap peas and cook for a further 3 minutes. Lift all the vegetables out with a slotted spoon, drain and refresh them under cold running water and set aside on a plate. Leave them to cool down while you prepare the fish fingers.

Pat the salmon dry with absorbent kitchen paper, roll it in the plate of seasoned flour, dip the salmon into the eggs and finally into the plate of sesame seeds. You can sprinkle more seeds over the fish if you like.

Toss the salad vegetables with the chopped tomatoes in their oil, lemon juice and chives and season with salt and pepper. Arrange the salad over a flat serving dish.

Now briefly heat the oil in a non-stick frying pan (skillet) over a high heat and fry the salmon fingers for about 2–3 minutes on each side, until the seeds are golden and the outer layers of fish are opaque. Lift the salmon fingers out and on to a plate covered with a thick layer of absorbent kitchen paper.

After a minute or two, arrange the salmon fingers diagonally across the salad, decorate with the wedges of lemon or lime and serve immediately. Squeeze either lemon or lime juice over your salmon and enjoy it while it is hot.

Prawn, Mango and Cucumber Salad

You can choose the type of prawns (shrimp) to suit your budget. Dill adds a mild aniseed tang, which contrasts well with the mango and cucumber. Radishes lose their pungency once cut, so prepare them at the last minute. The lime juice will enhance the sweetness of the radishes.

Serves 4

GF   **DF**   **RF**   **Q&E**

Dressing

Juice of 1 lime
1 teaspoon Dijon mustard*
1 tablespoon clear honey
3 tablespoons bottled fat-free French dressing or cold pressed extra virgin olive oil
Sea salt and freshly ground black pepper

Salad

1 ripe mango, peeled and stoned (pitted)
¾ cucumber, peeled
1 large bunch fresh radishes, trimmed
455g/16oz large king prawns (jumbo shrimp), peeled, heads and tails removed
15g/½oz fresh dill, finely chopped

* coeliacs please use gluten-free ingredients

First make the dressing: whisk together the lime juice, mustard, honey, French dressing or oil and season to taste.

Now make the salad. Cut the mango flesh into small chunks and thinly slice the cucumber. Arrange the cucumber slices in a ring on a large serving plate. Finely slice the radishes and combine them in a bowl with the prawns (shrimp) and mango chunks. Arrange this mixture in the centre and spoon over the dressing. Sprinkle with dill and serve immediately or keep chilled until needed.

Vegetarian Main Courses ...

Roasted Vegetable, Chestnut and Polenta Tarts

Roast chestnuts give this special Christmas treat for vegetarians a lovely festive feel. You can make the tarts any time of year if you use canned chestnuts or shelled pecan nuts. If there are more than three vegetarians then double or treble the quantities accordingly.

GF   DF   V

Serves 3

Pastry

115g/1 cup wheat-free flour mix*

30g/1oz organic butter or dairy-free margarine

30g/1oz hard white vegetable shortening (Trex or Cookeen are good)

1 organic free-range egg

A little cold filtered water

Filling

2 tablespoons cold pressed extra virgin olive oil

455g/1lb diced mixed root vegetables, such as parsnip, sweet potato and carrots or other favourites (once peeled and diced they should weigh about 340g/12oz)

100g/3½oz peeled whole chestnuts (frozen, canned and drained or vacuum packed)

1 tablespoon runny honey

Fresh thyme and a few sprigs to garnish

Sea salt and freshly ground black pepper

55g/⅓ cup quick-cook polenta

30g/1oz organic butter or dairy-free margarine and extra for glazing

Cayenne pepper

3 individual flan or tart tins (pans) or rings, plain or fluted, greased and floured

*** coeliacs please use gluten-free ingredients**

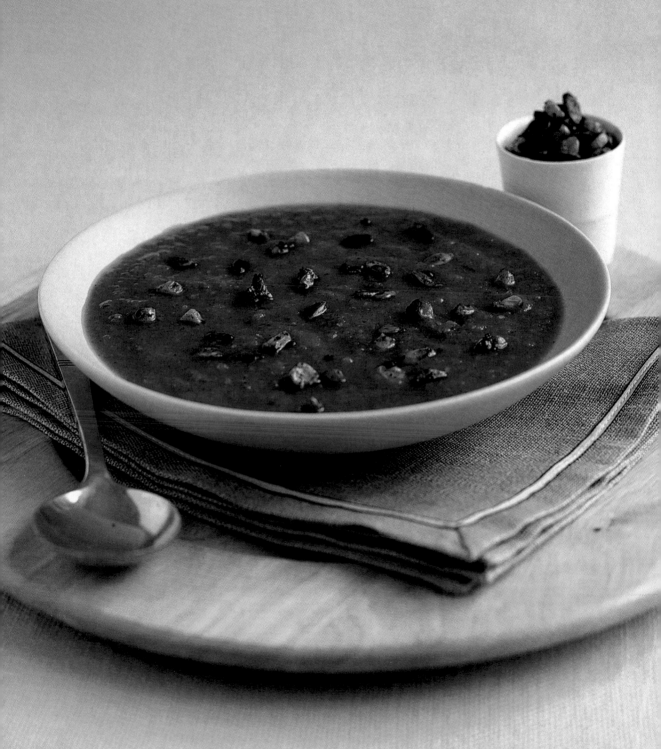

Pumpkin Soup with Creole Seeds (page 28)

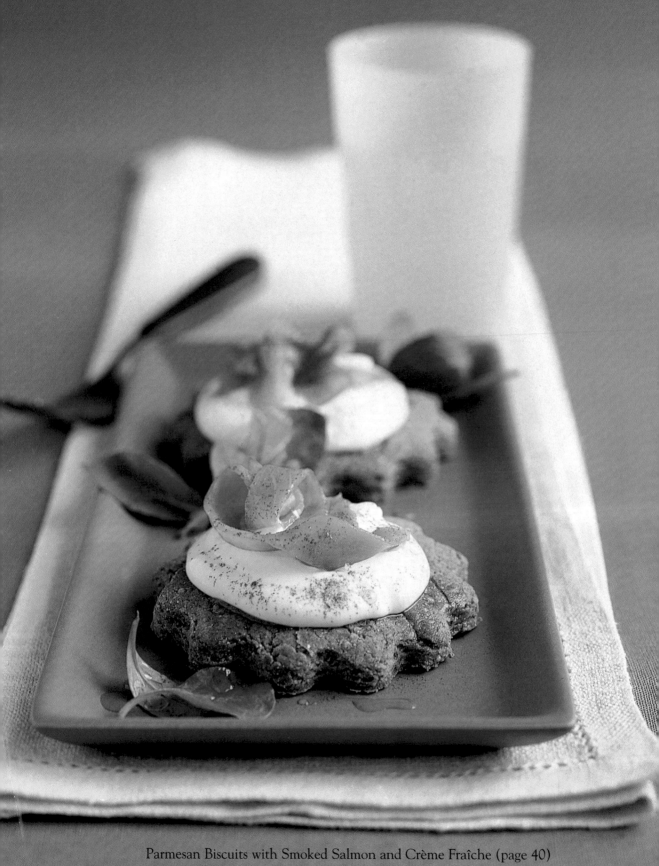

Parmesan Biscuits with Smoked Salmon and Crème Fraîche (page 40)

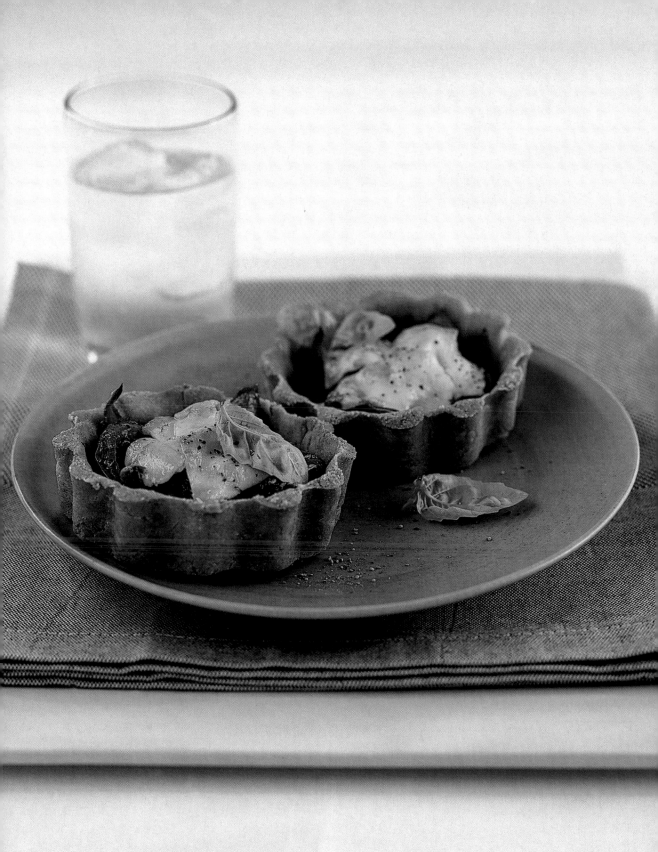

Tomato and Pesto Tarts (page 50)

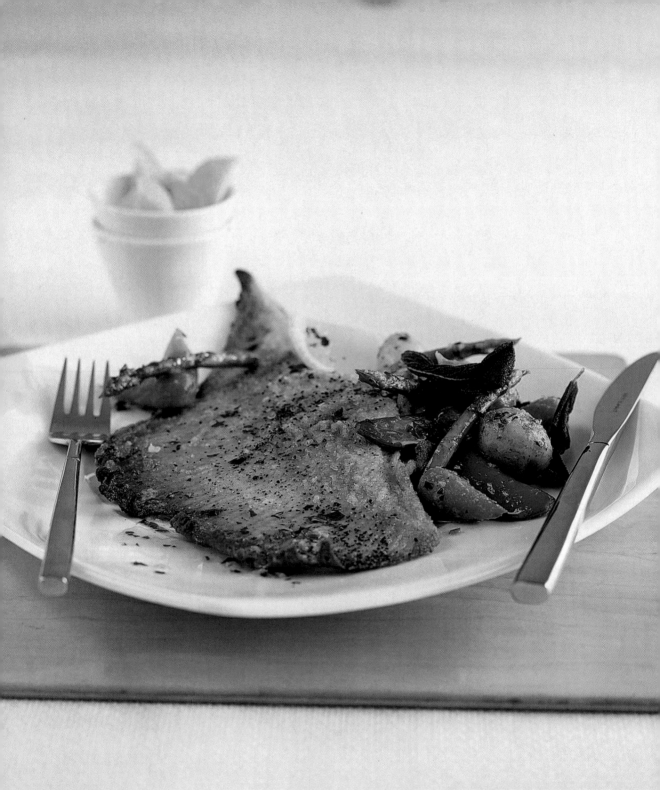

Roast Skate with Baby Summer Vegetables (page 58)

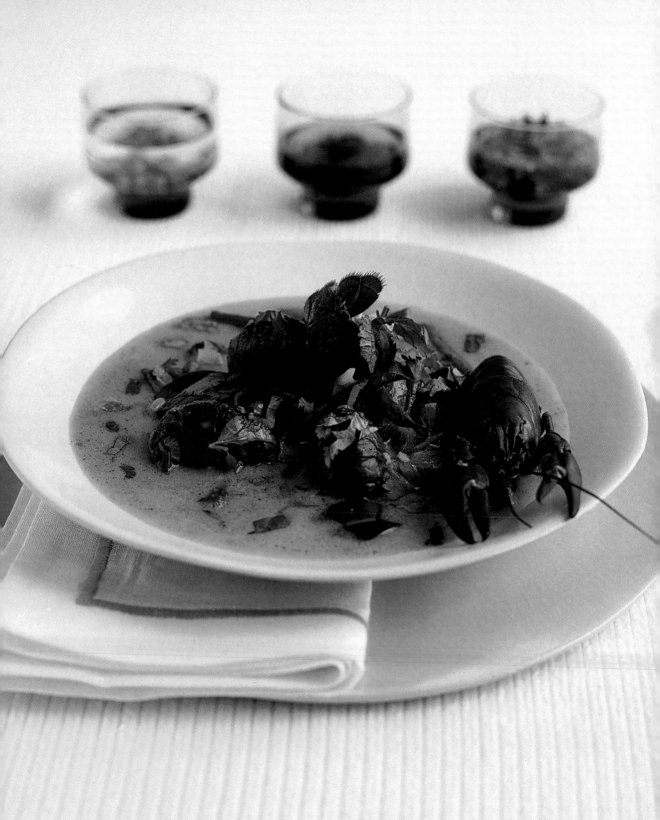

Thai Seafood Casserole (page 63)

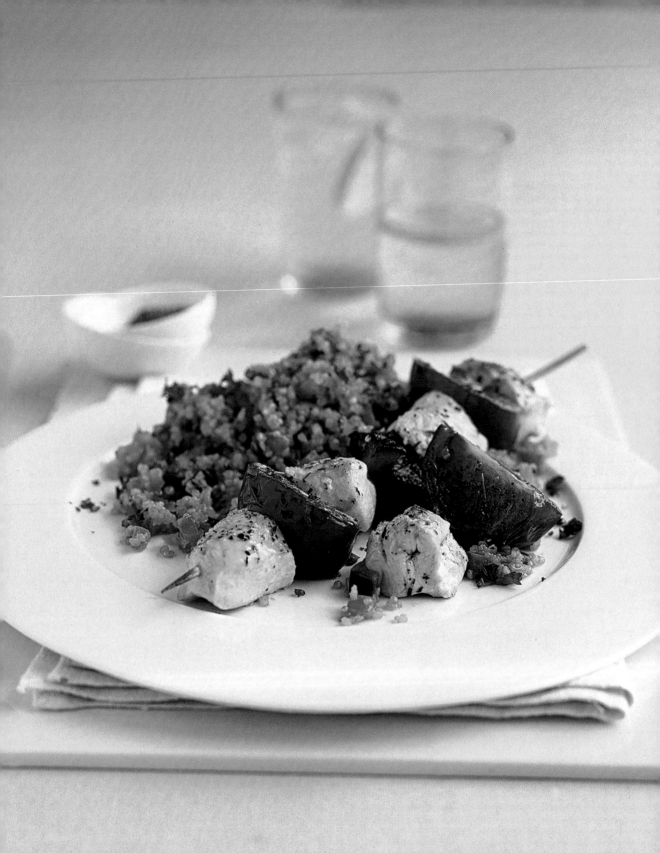

Chicken Kebabs with Quinoa Couscous (page 108)

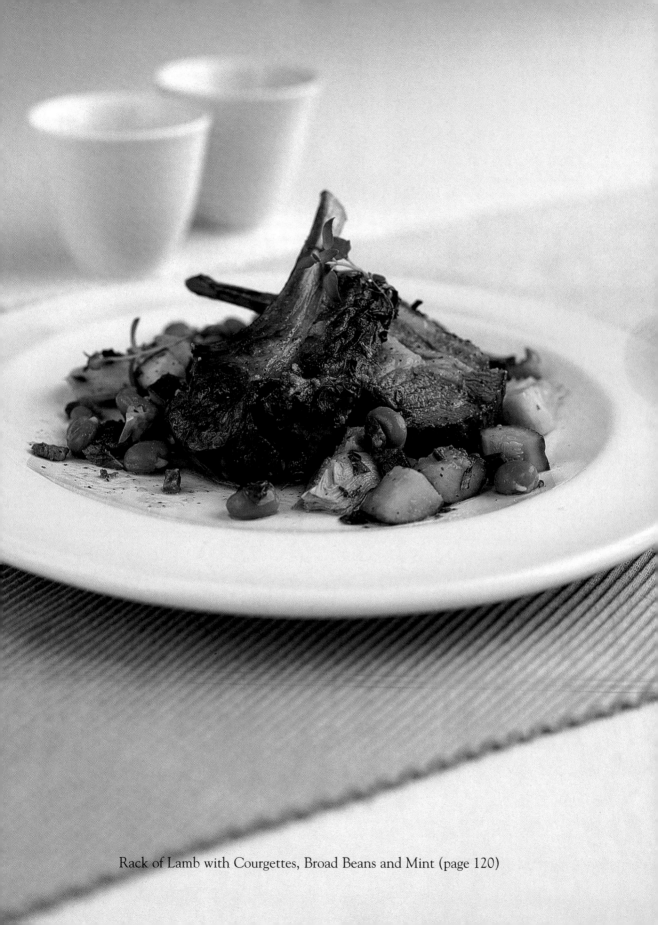

Rack of Lamb with Courgettes, Broad Beans and Mint (page 120)

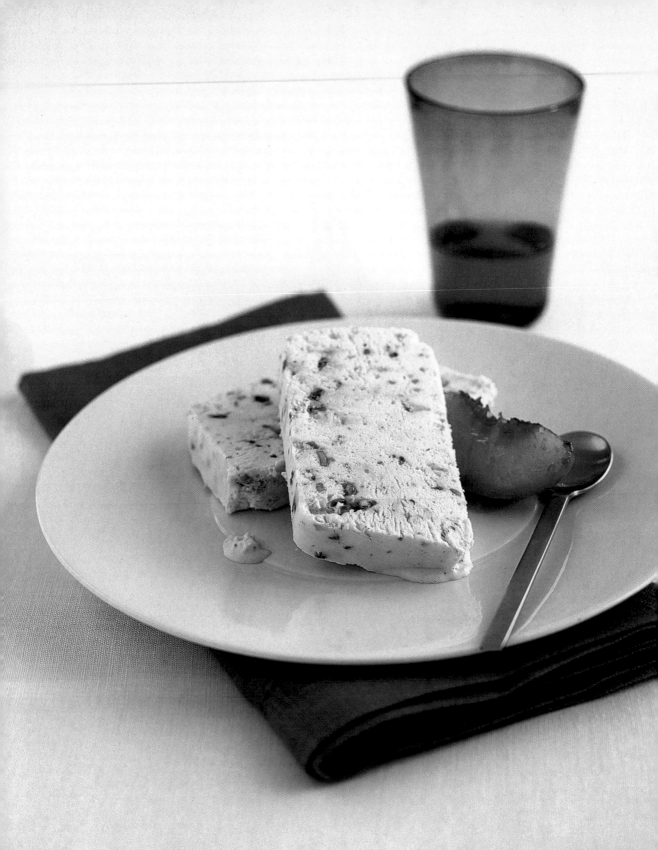

Pine Nut Semifreddo (page 210)

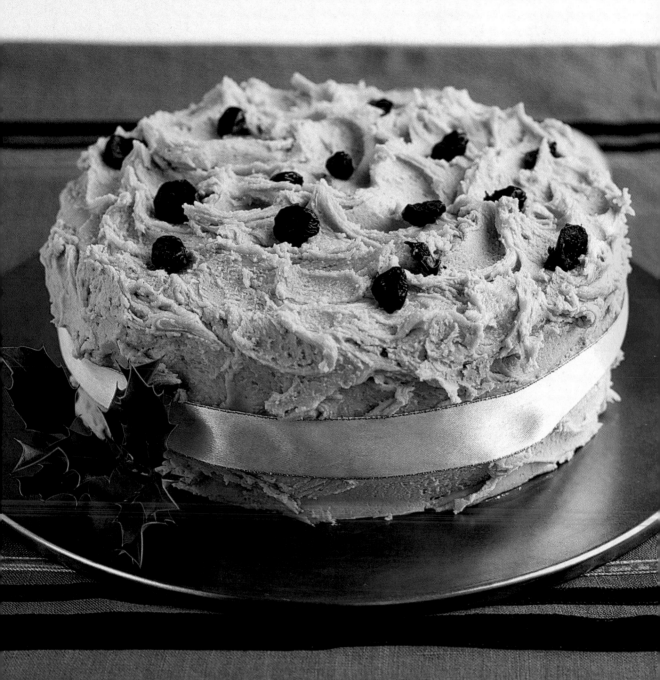

Creole Christmas Cake (page 252)

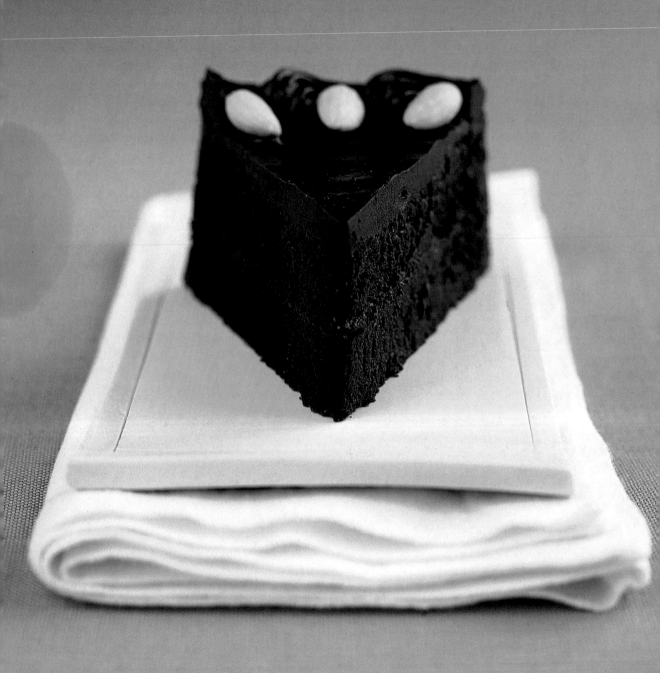

Chocolate Almond Gâteau (page 258)

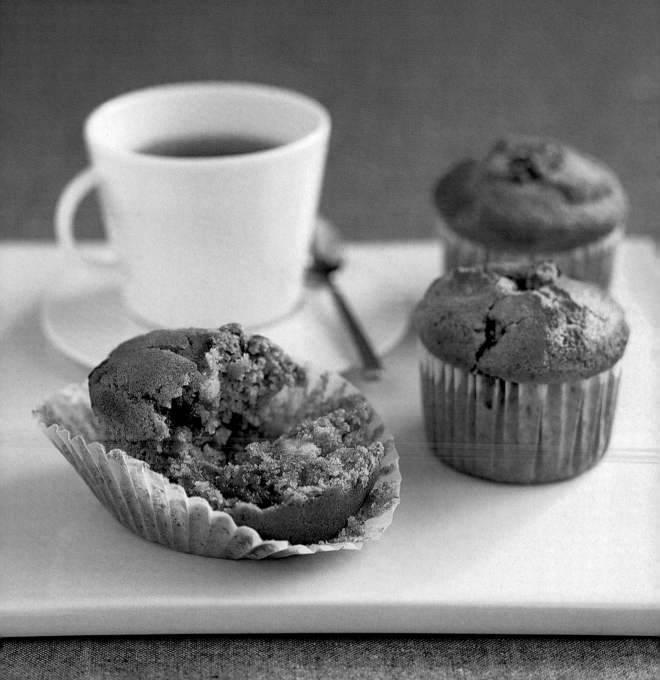

Raspberry and White Chocolate Muffins (page 270)

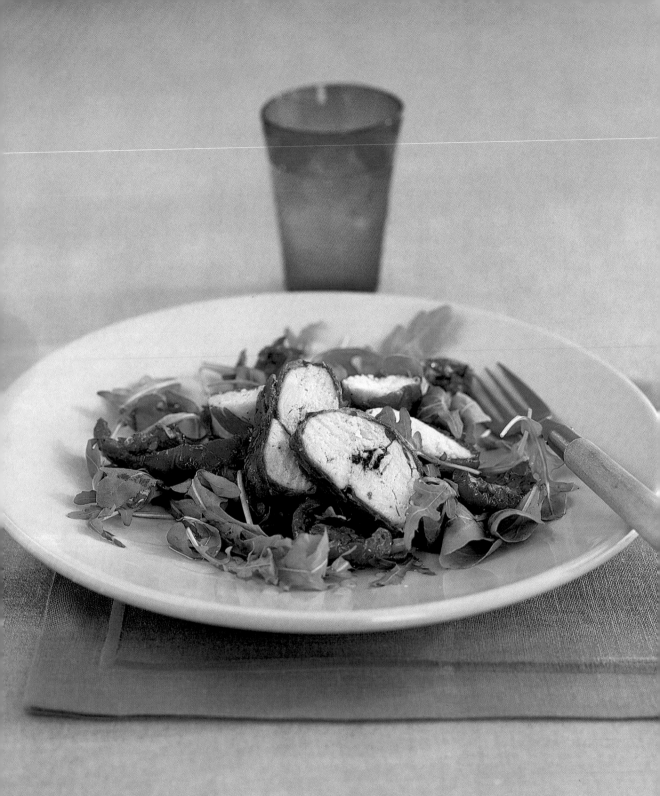

Chicken Kiev in Parma Ham (page 119)

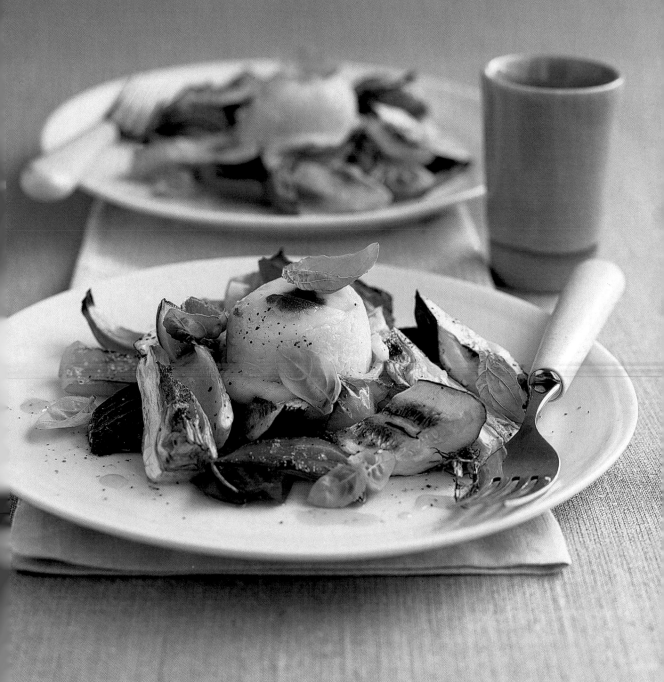

Roasted Vegetable and Goats' Cheese Salad (page 136)

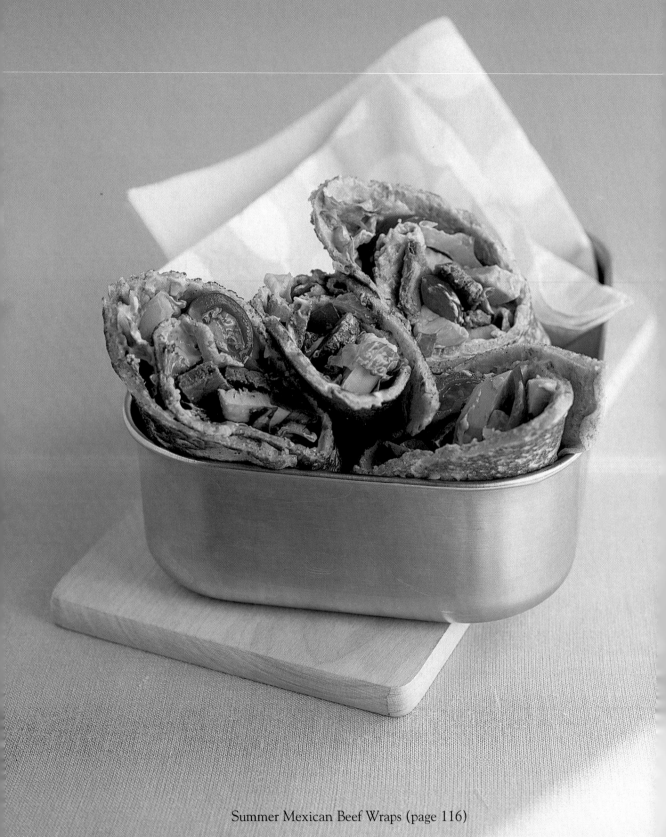

Summer Mexican Beef Wraps (page 116)

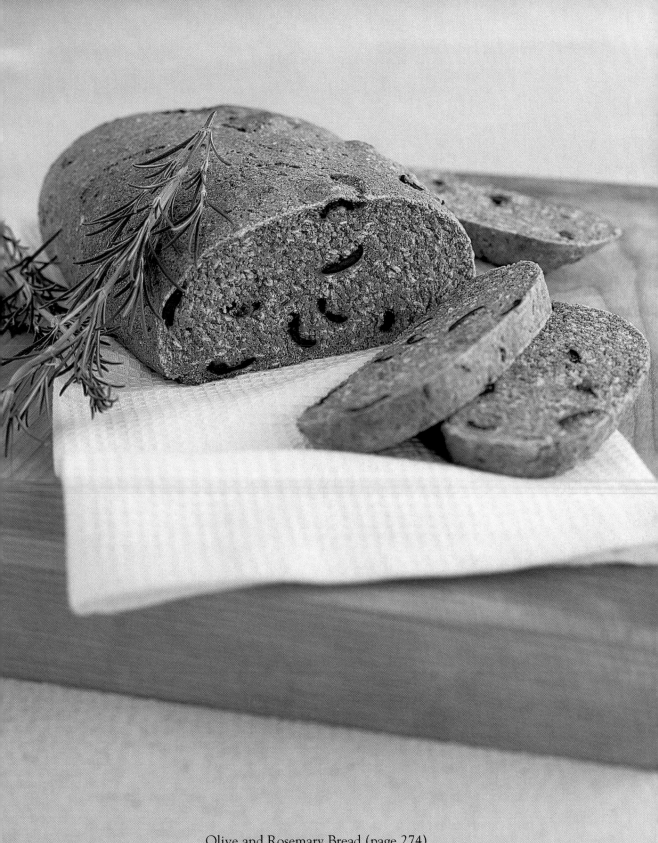

Olive and Rosemary Bread (page 274)

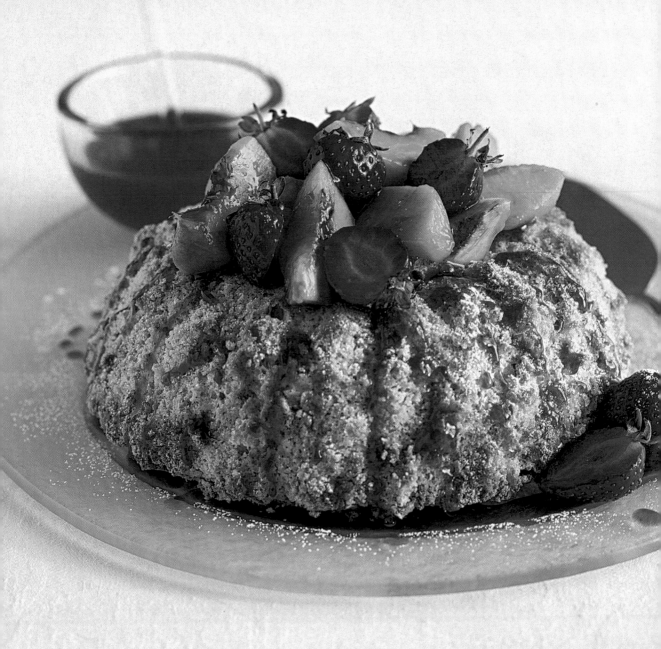

Peach Angel Ring with Strawberry Coulis (page 230)

Preheat the oven to 200°C/400°F/Gas mark 6.

Make the pastry first. Mix the flour, butter or dairy-free margarine and vegetable shortening in a food processor until the mixture resembles breadcrumbs. Add the egg and a little water at a time and mix until the dough comes together in a ball. Wrap the dough in clingfilm (plastic wrap) and chill for 30 minutes.

Meanwhile, make the filling. Heat the oil in a non-stick frying pan (skillet) and sauté the vegetables until softened. Stir in the chestnuts, honey, thyme, salt and pepper and continue to cook until the vegetables are tinged with gold.

Combine the polenta with 200ml/¾ cup of boiling filtered water in a small non-stick pan over moderate heat. Add the butter, salt, pepper and cayenne and cook for 2–3 minutes, beating until thick and creamy.

Roll the pastry out on a floured board and cut out 3 circles to fit the prepared tart tins (pans). I use 13cm/5in coffee saucers to cut around. Line each one with the pastry and neaten the edges. Fill each tart with a layer of baking parchment (wax paper) and ceramic baking beans and bake the tarts blind for about 10 minutes. Remove the tarts from the oven and carefully lift out the paper and beans. Return the tarts to the oven and bake for 5 minutes or until pale gold.

Take the tarts out of the oven and fill each one with the creamed polenta. Spoon the chestnut and vegetable mixture over the polenta and bake the tarts in the oven for about 10 minutes. Serve each one decorated with a sprig of thyme.

Caramelized Onion and Blue Cheese Pizza

If you are always short of time, you can buy wheat- or gluten-free pizza bases either by mail order (and freeze them) or from good health food stores or the 'well-being' sections of the big superstores. Alternatively, you can make your own yeast- and wheat-free pizza at home – it's much quicker to make than the yeast-based variety that take hours to prove and rise.

Makes 2 large pizzas

GF   V   Q&E

2 x Antoinette Savill Signature Series pizza bases (see page 304 for stockist) or

Pizza bases

450g/4 generous cups wheat-free white flour mix*

1 teaspoon unrefined golden caster (superfine) sugar

1 heaped teaspoon bicarbonate of soda (baking soda)

1 teaspoon sea salt

About 500–600ml/2–2⅓ cups buttermilk (depending on flour absorbency)

Topping

2 tablespoons olive oil, plus extra for drizzling

2 large red onions, very finely sliced

1 tablespoon unrefined golden caster (superfine) sugar

2 teaspoons balsamic vinegar

400g/14oz can chopped tomatoes

2 heaped tablespoons tomato purée (paste)

2 teaspoons dried oregano leaves

Freshly ground black pepper

4 heaped tablespoons crumbled or coarsely chopped organic blue cheese or dairy-free grated Cheddar-style cheese or mozzarella-style slices (see page 305 for stockist)

1 heaped tablespoon pine nuts

Preheat the oven to 230°C/450°F/Gas mark 8.

Heat the oil in a non-stick frying pan (skillet), add the onions and cook over medium heat until soft. Stir in the sugar and vinegar and cook until golden and caramelized.

Meanwhile, make the pizza bases. Sift the dry ingredients into a bowl, make a well and pour in 500ml/2 cups of buttermilk. Add more if necessary to bring the mixture together into a soft but not wet or sticky dough.

Turn the dough onto a floured board, knead briefly for a few seconds to tidy it up, then roll out into 2 × 25.5cm/10in rounds. Using a sharp knife, trim the edges to give a smooth, neat line. Place the bases on baking trays.

In a bowl, mix the canned tomatoes with the tomato purée (paste), oregano and pepper and spread the mixture evenly over each pizza base, going right up to the edges. Arrange the onions over the top of the tomato mixture then scatter the cheese all over each pizza and sprinkle with the pine nuts.

Drizzle with a little extra oil and bake for about 15 minutes until the pizzas are golden and bubbling.

If using the ready-made pizza bases simply top them in the same way and bake for the same amount of time.

Crème Fraîche and Sun-Dried Tomato Penne

This is the easiest of pasta dishes and it can be served simply with a big green salad of chicory, frisée and plenty of fresh basil.

Serves 6

GF   DF   V   Q&E

500g/1lb 2oz packet wheat-free penne*
250ml/1 cup half fat crème fraîche or dairy-free Tofutti Sour Supreme (see page 305 for stockist)
Sea Salt and freshly ground black pepper
100g/3½oz packet sun-dried tomatoes or sunblush tomatoes, drained of excess oil and cut into strips
3 heaped tablespoons tomato purée (paste)

Optional to serve
Grated pecorino cheese or Florentino Parmazano dairy-free alternative (see page 306 for stockist)

---

* coeliacs please use gluten-free ingredients

Bring a pan of salted water to the boil, add the pasta and cook until softened, stirring and separating the pasta from time to time. Drain the pasta and refresh with cold water. Refill the pan with salted water, bring it to the boil and cook the pasta until soft, stirring from time to time. (This method prevents the pasta becoming sticky.)

Meanwhile, mix the crème fraîche or Sour Supreme, salt and pepper, tomatoes and purée (paste) together in a big serving bowl. Drain the pasta, toss in the sauce and serve immediately, with or without a bowl of grated cheese.

Fettuccini with Rocket Pesto

You can make the pesto up to a week in advance, if you keep it sealed and chilled in the refrigerator. Bring the pesto back to room temperature before using. For a more substantial non-vegetarian meal you can serve this dish with grilled chicken, salmon, pork fillets or prawns (shrimp).

Serves 4

GF   DF   V   Q&E

Pesto

Sea salt and freshly ground black pepper

55g/⅓ cup pine nuts

55g/2oz fresh wild rocket (arugula), stalks included

1 garlic clove, peeled and coarsely chopped

55g/2oz freshly grated Parmesan or pecorino cheese or use dairy-free Florentino Parmazano (see page 306 for stockist)

1 tablespoon fresh lemon juice

8 tablespoons cold pressed extra virgin olive oil

455g/1lb Orgran gluten-free rice and corn fettuccini (see page 305 for stockist)

Place the pesto ingredients in a food processor and whiz briefly until the sauce is smooth. Do not over-blend or you will ruin the nutty texture.

Bring a pan of salted water to the boil, cook the fettuccini until softened, stirring and separating the pasta from time to time. Drain the pasta and refresh with cold water. Refill the pan with salted water, bring it to the boil and cook the pasta until soft, stirring from time to time. (This method prevents the pasta becoming sticky.)

Drain the fettuccini and toss in a warm serving bowl with the rocket (arugula) pesto.

Tagliatelle with Dolcelatte and Walnut Sauce

This pasta dish has a very rich and creamy sauce that partners well with a crisp chicory and frisée salad. For a fresh and crunchy texture use fresh walnuts, not ones that have been languishing in your store cupboard for months.

GF   V   Q&E

Serves 2

170g/6oz gluten-free tagliatelle (any brand)
125ml/½ cup organic single cream
100g/3½oz piece organic Dolcelatte cheese, crumbled or cubed (do not use strong cheeses such as Stilton)
55g/½ cup walnut pieces
Sea salt and freshly ground black pepper
1 heaped tablespoon torn fresh basil leaves

Bring a pan of salted water to the boil, add the pasta and cook until softened, stirring and separating the pasta from time to time. Drain the pasta and refresh with cold water. Refill the pan with salted water, bring it to the boil and cook the pasta until soft, stirring from time to time. (This method prevents the pasta becoming sticky.)

Meanwhile, gently heat the cream and cheese together in a small non-stick pan over moderate heat. Keep stirring the sauce so that it does not stick to the pan. As soon as it is melted and smooth, add the walnuts and season to taste with salt and pepper.

Drain the pasta and toss in a warm serving bowl with the sauce. Sprinkle with the basil and serve.

Cheese Croquettes

This is such a good way to use up old leftover bits of cheese as it makes a cheap and delicious meal, served either with a salad or with baked potatoes and green vegetables. Serve with tomato ketchup, salsa or relish*.

Serves 4

GF   V   Q&E

Croquettes

170g/6oz organic extra mature Cheddar cheese or any local hard cheeses such as Cheshire, Caerphilly, Wensleydale or others, grated

225g/generous 2 cups fresh wheat-free breadcrumbs*, crusts removed

½ small onion, grated

1 heaped tablespoon finely chopped parsley

1 heaped tablespoon finely chopped chives

1 heaped teaspoon mustard*

1 large organic free-range egg, lightly beaten

Sea salt and freshly ground black pepper

1 tablespoon Worcestershire sauce*

A little organic milk

To coat

2 organic free-range eggs, beaten

115g/1¼ cups fine, dry wheat-free breadcrumbs* or use Orgran gluten-free all-purpose crumbs (see page 305 for stockist)

Extra virgin olive oil for frying

* coeliacs please use gluten-free ingredients

Put all the croquette ingredients in a bowl and lightly mix together using your fingertips. Add extra Worcestershire sauce and a little more milk if the mixture is dry. Transfer to a food processor and whiz until it becomes a fine and solid mixture.

Put the beaten egg on one plate and the fine crumbs on another. Mould pieces of the croquette mixture into little cocktail-size sausages. Dip each one first in the egg and then in the breadcrumbs, pressing firmly so that the coating sticks.

Heat enough oil to shallow fry the croquettes in a non-stick frying pan (skillet) over medium heat. Fry the croquettes in batches until they are very hot all the way through, golden and crisp. Drain the croquettes on kitchen paper and serve immediately.

Broccoli and Blue Cheese Tart

I love the combination of broccoli and cheese and often have it with pasta, as a soup or as a soufflé. This tart can be made with any hard cheese you like and you can use half-fat crème fraîche to reduce the calories.

Serves 8   GF   V

Pastry

255g/9oz wheat-free flour mix*

130g/4½oz organic butter

1 large organic free-range egg

Cold filtered water

Filling

225g/8oz broccoli, cut into bite-sized florets

1 medium onion, finely sliced

3 tablespoons olive oil

1 garlic clove, crushed

½ teaspoon dried thyme

130g/4½oz piece pungent organic blue cheese, such as Gorgonzola or Roquefort, crumbled

200ml/¾ cup organic crème fraîche

4 large organic free-range eggs, beaten

Sea salt and freshly ground black pepper

Freshly grated Parmesan cheese

Optional

A sprinkling of cayenne pepper

30.5cm/11in non-stick, fluted, loose-bottomed flan ring, lined with a circle of baking parchment (wax paper) or Bake-O-Glide

* coeliacs please use gluten-free ingredients

Preheat the oven to 200°C/400°F/Gas mark 6.

Make the pastry first. Mix the flour and butter together in a food processor until they resemble crumbs. Add the egg and a pinch of salt and whiz briefly before adding a little water, then whiz until the mixture comes into a ball of dough. Wrap the dough in clingfilm (plastic wrap) and chill for 30 minutes.

Meanwhile, make the filling. Cook the broccoli until tender, drain, refresh under cold running water and leave to one side. While the broccoli is cooking, fry the onion in the oil over moderate heat until softened. Add the garlic and thyme and cook until the onions are tinged with gold.

Add the broccoli to the onions and gently stir in the cheese and crème fraîche. Remove from the heat, stir in the beaten eggs and season to taste with salt and pepper.

Roll the pastry out thinly, carefully line the prepared flan ring with it and neaten the edges.

Spoon the filling mixture into the pastry base and sprinkle with the Parmesan and cayenne. Bake in the oven for about 25 minutes until the pastry is golden and filling is set.

Torta di Risotto

You can prepare this dish in the morning, leave it in the refrigerator and bake it 40 minutes before sitting down to dinner. I serve Torta di Risotto with a mixed green salad and the bean salad recipe on page 137.

If you are not a great fan of courgettes (zucchini), you can use aubergines (eggplant) instead but you will need more oil to cook them.

GF   V

Serves 4–6

1½ medium-sized courgettes (zucchini), trimmed, halved across and cut into thin slices lengthways – discard the tough outer slices

4 tablespoons cold pressed extra virgin olive oil

2 garlic cloves, crushed

400g/14oz can chopped tomatoes

1 teaspoon balsamic vinegar

1 heaped teaspoon unrefined golden granulated sugar

1 teaspoon dried chopped sage leaves

Sea salt and freshly ground black pepper

255g/9oz Arborio risotto rice

About 250ml/1 cup hot filtered water or allergy-free vegetable stock (bouillon)

2 tablespoons Orgran all purpose crumbs (see page 305 for stockist) or very fine homemade gluten-free breadcrumbs

100g/3½oz piece organic extra strong/mature Cheddar or an Italian hard cheese, cubed

30g/1oz piece fresh Parmesan cheese, finely grated

130g/4½oz organic mozzarella cheese, drained and cubed

Preheat the oven to 220°C/425°F/Gas mark 7.

Fry the courgette (zucchini) slices in 2 tablespoons of the oil in a frying pan (skillet) until soft and golden brown. Meanwhile, heat the remaining oil in another pan and briefly cook the garlic over medium heat. Stir in the tomatoes, vinegar, sugar, sage, salt and pepper and simmer for a couple of minutes. Stir in the rice and the water or stock (bouillon). Simmer at bubbling point until the rice is tender, stirring regularly, and adding a little more water or stock (bouillon) as necessary.

Lightly oil a standard-sized, non-stick loaf tin (pan) and sprinkle all over the base and sides with 1 tablespoon of crumbs. Shake the excess into a small saucer.

Stir the cheeses into the risotto and spoon half the mixture over the base of the tin (pan). Arrange the courgette (zucchini) slices in overlapping rows along the rice and cover with the remaining risotto. Sprinkle the remaining crumbs over the top and bake in the oven for about 35 minutes until golden and bubbling.

Let the torta stand for 10 minutes, then run a long-bladed knife between it and the tin (pan) and invert the torta onto a flat, warm serving dish. Tap the tin (pan) until you can lift it off. Serve immediately, cutting the torta into thick slices so that it holds its shape.

Vegetable, Cheese and Onion Pie

This hearty pie is a very economical way of feeding the family in mid-winter, when everyone needs warm and comforting food. You can, if you wish, add chopped chicken or turkey meat if you have some leftover from a Sunday roast.

Serves 4–6

GF **DF** **V**

Pastry

100g/¾ cup organic rice flour
100g/¾ cup Orgran self-raising flour (see page 305 for stockist)
55g/2oz organic butter or dairy-free margarine
55g/2oz white vegetable shortening (Trex or Cookeen are good)
1 large organic free-range egg, beaten
Cold filtered water

Filling

170g/6oz each carrots, swede and parsnip, peeled and cut into bite-size chunks
340g/12oz prepared leeks, chopped into bite-size chunks
55g/2oz organic butter or dairy-free margarine
55g/scant ½ cup wheat-free flour mix*
800ml/3 cups organic milk or organic dairy-free unsweetened soya milk
1 heaped teaspoon Dijon mustard*
1 tablespoon Worcestershire sauce*
Sea salt and freshly ground black pepper
A little freshly grated nutmeg
115g/4oz any organic hard cheese, crumbled, or dairy-free Redwoods grated Cheddar-style cheese (see page 305 for stockist)

* coeliacs please use gluten-free ingredients

Make the pastry first. Mix the flours, butter or margarine and the shortening in a food processor until the mixture resembles crumbs. Add three-quarters of the egg and a little water at a time and process until the mixture comes together into a ball of dough. Wrap the dough in clingfilm (plastic wrap) and chill for half an hour while you prepare the filling.

Cook all the root vegetables together in a pan of boiling water for a few minutes, then add the leeks and cook until soft. Drain the vegetables and refresh them under cold running water.

While the vegetables are cooking, make the white sauce. Melt the butter or margarine in a non-stick pan over moderate heat and then stir in the flour. Gradually beat in the milk until you have a smooth sauce. Season the sauce with the mustard, Worcestershire sauce, salt, pepper and grated nutmeg. Stir the vegetables into the sauce and mix in the crumbled or grated cheese. Transfer the mixture into a deep pie dish. Brush the edges of the dish with cold filtered water.

Roll the pastry out on a floured board until it is big enough to cover the pie dish with about 1cm/½ in overhanging. Lift the pastry onto the pie dish and, using your fingers, crimp the edges all round the pie into a fluted edge. Brush the pastry with the remaining beaten egg, cut a small hole in the centre of the pastry so that the steam can escape and bake in the oven for about 35 minutes until the pastry is golden and the filling is bubbling.

Wild Mushroom Tortelli

This is a sophisticated dish that is delicious in the autumn (fall) when the mushrooms are gathered from the woods and fields. At other times of the year you can use the cultivated 'wild' mushrooms found in good supermarkets or you can mix standard cultivated mushrooms with a handful of dried wild mushrooms.

GF   DF   V   Q&E

Serves 4

340g/12oz Orgran gluten-free tortelli (pasta shapes) (see page 305 for stockist)
255g/9oz cultivated mushrooms, wiped clean, trimmed if necessary and sliced
155g/5½oz fresh wild mushrooms
55g/2oz organic butter or dairy-free margarine
1 garlic clove, crushed
340g/12oz tub dairy-free Tofutti Sour Supreme (see page 305 for stockist)
30g/1oz Parmesan or dairy-free Florentino Parmazano (see page 306 for stockist)
Sea salt and freshly ground black pepper
2 tablespoons chopped fresh parsley

Optional
Extra Parmesan or dairy-free cheese to serve

Cook the tortelli in a pan of salted boiling water until softened, stirring and separating the pasta from time to time. Drain the pasta and refresh with cold water. Refill the pan with salted water, bring it to the boil and cook the pasta until soft, stirring from time to time. (This method prevents the pasta becoming sticky.)

Meanwhile, sauté the mushrooms in the butter or margarine in a non-stick frying pan (skillet), over moderate heat, until tinged with gold and softened. Stir in the garlic and cook for a couple of minutes. Stir in the Sour Supreme and cheese, season to taste and keep warm while you drain the cooked pasta.

Put the drained pasta into a warm bowl, spoon the sauce over and toss briefly before sprinkling with the parsley. Serve immediately with extra cheese if desired.

Quinoa Risotto

This recipe is a very quick, easy and nutritious version of the traditional risotto but it does need a very high quality pesto, or you can make your own dairy- or nut-free version according to dietary needs.

Serves 2

GF   V   Q&E

130g/¾ cup quinoa, thoroughly rinsed in cold running water
500ml/2 cups cold filtered water
225g/8oz button mushrooms, wiped clean
2 tablespoons of oil drained from the sunblush tomatoes or use cold pressed extra virgin olive oil
85g/2½oz (drained weight) sunblush tomatoes, coarsely chopped
1 small garlic clove, crushed
A large pinch of sea salt and freshly ground black pepper
2 tablespoons fresh deli-made pesto or organic pesto

Optional
Grated Parmesan or pecorino cheese

Put the quinoa in a pan with the water and bring to the boil over medium heat. Stir from time to time to prevent the quinoa sticking. Meanwhile, fry the mushrooms in a non-stick pan with the 2 tablespoons of oil until golden. Stir in the tomatoes and garlic, season with salt and pepper and cook for about 5 minutes.

When the quinoa has doubled in size and is translucent, stir in the mushroom mixture and pesto, adjust the seasoning and serve immediately with the cheese.

Mushroom and Garlic Roulade

Roulades are so easy to make and ideal for picnics and buffets. We often have this one for lunch with a mixed salad and baby new potatoes. Any leftovers last brilliantly for a couple of days in the refrigerator.

Serves 6–8

GF   DF   V

Flavoured milk

580ml/2¼ cups organic milk or organic unsweetened dairy-free soya milk

½ onion, halved and studded with 4 cloves

1 celery stick, cut into 3 pieces

1 bay leaf and a few stalks of parsley

A good pinch of sea salt

10 black peppercorns

Roulade

455g/1lb mushrooms, wiped clean

85g/3oz organic butter or dairy-free margarine

85g/¾ cup wheat-free flour mix*

4 large organic free-range eggs, separated

Sea salt and freshly ground black pepper

Freshly grated nutmeg

Filling

395g/14oz reduced-fat cream cheese or Tofutti Creamy Smooth dairy-free alternative (see page 305 for stockist)

2 heaped tablespoons chopped fresh parsley, chives or coriander (cilantro)

A little organic milk or unsweetened organic dairy-free soya milk

33 x 39cm/12 x 14in Swiss roll tin (pan) lined with non-stick baking parchment (wax paper)

* coeliacs please use gluten-free ingredients

The Big Book of Wheat-Free Cooking

Preheat the oven to 220°C/425°F/Gas mark 7.

Put all the ingredients for the flavoured milk in a pan and bring to just below boiling point. Remove from the heat and leave to infuse for 45 minutes then strain the milk and leave to one side.

Blend the mushrooms in a food processor then transfer to a sieve lined with a treble thickness of absorbent kitchen paper and leave to one side.

Meanwhile, melt the butter or margarine in a pan over low heat and stir in the flour. Cook for a couple of minutes then gradually stir in the flavoured milk and cook until the sauce boils. Remove from the heat and stir the egg yolks into the sauce one by one. Season with salt, pepper and nutmeg.

Now fold in the raw mushrooms. Whisk the egg whites until stiff and fold these into the mushroom mixture. Pour the mixture into the prepared tin (pan) and bake for about 20–25 minutes until the roulade feels just firm to the touch.

Remove the roulade from the oven and cover with baking parchment (wax paper) and a clean, damp cloth until cool.

To make the filling, blend the ingredients together in a small bowl, using a wooden spoon, until you have a spreadable mixture.

To assemble the roulade, remove the paper and cloth and put a fresh sheet of the parchment (wax paper) onto a clean surface. Invert the roulade onto this and carefully peel off the paper lining. Spread the roulade with the cream cheese mixture and roll it up lengthways like a Swiss roll. Slide onto a serving dish and serve in slices.

Broccoli and Toasted Breadcrumb Penne

You don't need much pasta for this dish and you can use whatever shape you like. Alternatively, you can increase the amount of pasta and decrease both the broccoli and the crumbs. Serve with a mixed salad with plenty of fresh herbs.

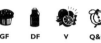

Serves 2

115g/4oz wheat-free pasta* (shells, bows, twists or tubes are all good)
Sea salt and freshly ground black pepper
2 tablespoons cold pressed extra virgin olive oil, plus more for drizzling
85g/3oz wheat-free breadcrumbs*
1 garlic clove, crushed
30g/1oz Parmesan, finely grated or dairy-free Florentino Parmazano (see page 306 for stockist)
225g/8oz fresh broccoli, trimmed into bite-size florets
Juice of 1 small lemon

Optional

Extra Parmesan or Parmazano to serve

* coeliacs please use gluten-free ingredients

Bring a pan of salted water to the boil and cook the pasta until softened, stirring and separating the pasta from time to time. Drain the pasta and refresh with cold water. Refill the pan with salted water, bring it to the boil and cook the pasta until soft, stirring from time to time. (This method prevents the pasta becoming sticky.)

Meanwhile, heat the oil in a non-stick frying pan (skillet), add the breadcrumbs and fry until golden. Add the garlic and cheese and stir over medium heat for a couple of minutes until the breadcrumbs are dark gold. Transfer the crumbs to a warm serving bowl. Meanwhile, steam or boil the broccoli until cooked but still crunchy in the middle. Drain if necessary and toss the broccoli in the serving bowl with the other ingredients. Drain the pasta, toss with the broccoli mixture, sprinkle with the extra cheese, the lemon juice and pepper and serve immediately.

Winter Thai Stir-Fry

As you would if making a fresh salad, plan ahead to make sure that you have fresh and crisp ingredients for the stir-fry. This ensures that you get the maximum nutrients as well as the best flavours and textures.

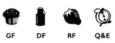

GF   DF   RF   Q&E

Serves 1

70g/1 cup thinly sliced red cabbage
60g/½ cup thinly cut carrot sticks
60g/¾ cup small broccoli florets
60g/¾ cup small cauliflower florets
60g/1 cup mung or bean sprouts (or any other fresh vegetables you have available)
1 tablespoon cold pressed extra virgin olive oil
½ garlic clove, crushed
½ small chilli (any strength), finely chopped, remove seeds for a milder taste
¼ teaspoon coriander seeds
1 heaped teaspoon grated root ginger
1 tablespoon soy sauce*
Sea salt and freshly ground black pepper
1 tablespoon chopped fresh coriander (cilantro) leaves

* coeliacs please use gluten-free ingredients

First, prepare all your vegetables. Heat the oil in the wok over a high heat.

Stir-fry the cabbage, carrots, broccoli, cauliflower and the remaining cup of your choice of vegetables together for 3 minutes. If your choice is bean sprouts or some other very fine vegetable, add them after 3 minutes along with the garlic, chilli, coriander seeds and ginger. Fry everything together for about another 2 minutes, by which time the bean sprouts will be cooked through too.

Toss the ingredients regularly to ensure that they cook evenly. Season with the soy sauce and pepper, sprinkle with the coriander (cilantro) leaves and serve immediately.

Feta, Courgette and Tomato Pizza

Here are two easy ways to conjure up a pizza: one is instant while the other takes a fraction more time but is, of course, fresher and even more delicious. You can put any topping you like on to this pizza base and be as extravagant (artichokes, asparagus, prawns or shrimp) or as economical (cheese and tomato) as you like. I find that half a pizza is enough for me, so we usually share one. If you are on your own, I suggest halving the pizza and freezing half for another time. Simply defrost it as usual and cook until piping hot.

INSTANT
PIZZA

Serves 1

GF   V   Q&E

Instant pizza

400g/14oz can ratatouille – a high quality brand will ensure lots of courgettes (zucchini)

1 small garlic clove, crushed

2 tablespoons tomato purée (paste)

Sea salt and freshly ground black pepper

Minced chilli in oil or freshly chopped chilli, according to taste

1 ready-made wheat-free pizza base* (see page 304 for stockist)

110g/4oz organic feta cheese, thinly sliced

Large pinch of herbes de Provence (mixed herbs can be used as an alternative)

Drizzle of cold pressed extra virgin olive oil

Super pizza

240g/8½oz sunblush tomatoes in olive oil, (available in Sainsbury's) drained, but keep the oil for later

1 small garlic clove, crushed

2 tablespoons tomato purée (paste)

Sea salt and freshly ground black pepper

Minced chilli or freshly chopped chilli, according to taste

1 ready-made wheat-free pizza base* (see page 304 for stockist)

1 small courgette (zucchini), finely sliced

110g/4oz organic feta cheese, thinly sliced

A large pinch of herbes de Provence (or mixed herbs)

* coeliacs please use gluten-free ingredients

Preheat the oven to 220°C/425°F/Gas mark 7.

To make the instant pizza, mix the ratatouille in a bowl with the garlic, tomato purée (paste), salt and pepper and chilli seasoning; spread the mixture over the pizza base and slide it on to a baking tray. Cover with the feta cheese, sprinkle liberally with the herbs and some more black pepper and drizzle with oil. Bake for 25 minutes or until bubbling and very hot.

To make the super pizza, mix the sunblush tomatoes in a bowl with the garlic, tomato purée (paste), salt and pepper and chilli seasoning; spread the mixture evenly over the pizza base, pressing it right to the edges. Slide it on to a baking tray.

Bring a pan of water to the boil and cook the courgettes (zucchini) for about 3 minutes or until they are just cooked but still crunchy. Drain and rinse under cold running water. Pat them dry in a double thickness of absorbent kitchen paper and then arrange the courgettes (zucchini) all over the pizza. Cover with the feta cheese, sprinkle liberally with the herbs and some more black pepper, and drizzle with some of the sunblush tomato oil. Bake for 25 minutes or until bubbling and very hot.

Griddled Sweet Potatoes with Three-Bean Salad

This recipe is a good filling and warming winter dish that is ideal for lunch or a light supper. You can use any of your favourite beans and mix and match your own combinations.

GF	DF	V	RF	Q&E

Serves 3

Potatoes

600g/1lb 5oz sweet potatoes (orange flesh), peeled and cut into 1.2 cm/½in thick slices
1 tablespoon cold pressed extra virgin olive oil

Bean salad

150g/scant 1 cup canned red kidney beans, drained and rinsed under cold water
150g/¾ cup canned butter (lima) beans, drained and rinsed under cold water
150g/scant 2 cups fine green beans, cut into thirds
Drizzle of bottled fat-free French dressing, or cold pressed extra virgin olive oil
Freshly ground black pepper
Sprinkling of chopped fresh parsley

Bring a pan of water to the boil, add the potato slices and cook for 5 minutes. Carefully lift them out with a slotted spoon or spatula and leave to drain. Heat the oil in a frying pan (skillet) over a high heat for a few seconds and then place the potato slices carefully in the pan. Season with a little pepper and sauté the potatoes until they are dark brown at the edges, golden in the middle and soft all the way through.

Meanwhile, make the salad. Rinse the kidney beans and butter (lima) beans under cold water and drain them. Bring a saucepan of water to the boil, add the green beans and cook them for 2 minutes so that they remain crunchy. Add the kidney beans and the butter (lima) beans to the pan and cook for 1 minute more. Drain all the beans in a colander, rinse them with warm water and drain again.

Put all the beans into a salad bowl, toss them in the dressing, season to taste with pepper and sprinkle with the fresh parsley. Serve the sauté potato slices in an overlapping circle in the centre of each plate, top with a mound of the bean salad and eat straightaway.

Lemon and Spinach Risotto

Cheap and easy recipes are indispensable, whether feeding the family or entertaining. This risotto is ideal for either scenario, and can be served with a big green and herb salad and a tomato and basil salad.

Serves 4

GF   DF   V   Q&E

75g/¼ cup organic butter or dairy-free margarine
1 tablespoon cold pressed extra virgin olive oil
1 onion, finely chopped
300g/1½ cups Arborio rice
1 litre/4 cups allergy-free vegetable stock (bouillon)
125g/4½oz fresh young spinach leaves, coarsely chopped
Finely grated rind and juice of 1 unwaxed lemon
60g/½ cup freshly grated reduced-fat hard cheese or dairy-free cheese (see page 305 for stockist)
Sea salt and freshly ground black pepper

Melt the margarine or butter with the oil in a large pan over a low heat and stir in the onions. Cook them until soft but do not let them brown. Add the rice, stir for about 30 seconds and then pour in the vegetable stock (bouillon). Simmer the rice until it is plump and soft, stirring regularly, adding more stock (bouillon) if needed.

Gently stir in the spinach, simmer for another couple of minutes until it has softened, and then stir in the lemon rind and juice, cheese, salt and pepper.

Serve the risotto immediately. If you want to reheat the risotto the next day, add some more stock (bouillon), lemon juice and a dash of oil and heat very gently, stirring constantly.

Fusilli with Roasted Vegetables and Olives

This easy pasta dish can be served hot or cold, and you can use any seasonal vegetables you like as long as they roast well. Other ideas are to use chopped aubergine (eggplant), French beans, squashes or baby carrots.

Serves 4–6

GF DF V

1 yellow pepper (bell pepper) and 1 green pepper (bell pepper), seeded and chopped into large pieces

2 small red onions, cut into 8 wedges

3 courgettes (zucchini), cut into about 8–10 diagonal chunks

4 vine tomatoes, stalks and tops removed

110–140g/4–5oz asparagus tips

5 tablespoons cold pressed extra virgin olive oil and 2 tablespoons extra virgin olive oil for tossing the pasta

1 heaped tablespoon chopped fresh rosemary leaves

255g/3 cups wheat-free fusilli pasta*

Sea salt and freshly ground black pepper

1 large garlic clove, crushed

85g/½ cup pitted black olives*

7g/¼oz fresh flat-leaf parsley, finely chopped

Optional
Minced chilli in oil, fresh chilli or chilli sauce*

* *coeliacs please use gluten-free ingredients*

The Big Book of Wheat-Free Cooking

Preheat the oven to 200°C/400°F/Gas mark 6.

Place all the vegetables in the oven's roasting tray or a big roasting pan, and sprinkle with the 5 tablespoons of olive oil. Make sure everything is evenly coated and then sprinkle over all the rosemary. Roast the vegetables in the oven for about 40 minutes until all the vegetables are cooked – some will be browned or crispy at the edges and some will just be softly cooked and glazed. I usually turn the tray around for more even baking but if you have a fan oven this shouldn't be necessary.

About halfway through the cooking time, bring a pan of water to the boil and add some salt. Cook the pasta according to the instructions until al dente. Drain the pasta, transfer to a serving bowl and toss in the 2 tablespoons of extra virgin olive oil. Season with salt, pepper, garlic, mix in the olives and add the chilli if you like your pasta spiced up.

As soon as the vegetables are ready, mix them into the pasta, sprinkle with fresh parsley and serve hot. Alternatively, wait for the mixture to cool, cover and chill until needed, but serve at room temperature.

Cheese Roulade with Walnuts

This is a brilliant vegetarian alternative to roast meats, game or turkey. We usually cook it during the Easter and Christmas periods, as it ensures that no vegetarians feel left out of the festivities.

This roulade works well when made a day in advance. Not only does it cut more easily, it also gives you more time to pamper yourself before friends or family arrive!

Serves 6

Roulade

30g/2 tablespoons dairy-free margarine or butter

30g/¼ cup wheat-free flour mix*

200ml/¾ cup skimmed milk

Sea salt and freshly ground black pepper

Freshly grated nutmeg

Pinch of cayenne pepper

4 large organic free-range eggs, separated

1 tablespoon of Dijon mustard*

85g/¾ cup grated reduced-fat hard cheese

60g/½ cup walnuts, very finely chopped, plus the same amount again for sprinkling on the non-stick paper

Filling

500g/2 cups virtually fat-free fromage frais

425g/15oz can artichoke hearts, well drained and thinly sliced

7g/¼oz chopped fresh parsley

33 x 23cm (13 x 9in) Swiss-roll/roulade tin (pan), lined with non-stick baking paper

1 large sheet of non-stick baking parchment (wax paper) sprinkled with 60g (½ cup) chopped walnuts, ready to turn the cooked roulade out immediately it comes out of the oven

* coeliacs please use gluten-free ingredients

Preheat the oven to 200°C/400°F/Gas mark 6.

Melt the margarine or butter in a small saucepan, stir in the flour and cook for a minute before gradually incorporating the milk. Let the mixture come to the boil, stirring all the time and cook for a couple of minutes. Remove it from the heat and season with salt, pepper, nutmeg and cayenne. Stir in the egg yolks, mustard, grated cheese and 60g/½ cup of walnuts.

In a large bowl, whisk the egg whites until stiff and then fold them into the cheese mixture. Gently pour and scrape the mixture into the prepared tin (pan) and bake in the oven for about 10–15 minutes, or until golden and firm to touch.

Turn the roulade out on to the walnut-sprinkled baking parchment (wax paper). The easiest way to do this is by flipping the roulade tin (pan) down on to the paper. Quickly peel the lining paper off the roulade and discard it. Cover with a clean cloth and leave to cool.

When cool, lift the cloth off the roulade and spread the roulade with the fromage frais. Now arrange the artichokes over the fromage frais, sprinkle the parsley over the artichokes, season with a little salt and plenty of pepper and roll up the roulade. Using the paper to help you, pull the roulade over a little at a time until it is completely rolled up. Keep it wrapped up securely in the paper and chill until needed.

Trim off the edges and serve the roulade cut into slices.

Asparagus and Spinach Picnic Tart

If you have a vegetable patch in your garden, you will probably agree that, amongst the plants that are classed as 'stalks and shoots', the undoubted aristocrat and noblest of them all is the asparagus. Its short season means that there is no time to get tired of this epicurean vegetable. This recipe makes a few stems go a long way.

Serves 6

GF   V

Pastry

255g/2¼ cups wheat-free flour mix*
125g/4½oz organic butter, cut into 8 pieces
1 large organic free-range egg
Pinch of sea salt
A little cold water

Filling

1 bundle asparagus, about 19 long spears, trimmed to fit into the pastry-lined baking tray
125g/4½oz fresh young spinach leaves, washed
250ml/1 cup reduced-fat crème fraîche
85g/¾ cup grated reduced-fat hard cheese
4 large organic free-range eggs, lightly beaten in a bowl
Freshly grated nutmeg
Sea salt and freshly ground black pepper
Pinch of cayenne pepper

ceramic baking beans
24cm/9½in square, loose-bottomed non-stick baking tray, lined with a square of non-stick baking parchment (wax paper)

* coeliacs please use gluten-free ingredients

Preheat the oven to 200°C/400°F/Gas mark 6.

Make the pastry by briefly blending all the ingredients, except the water, in a food processor until it resembles breadcrumbs. Now add a little water and whizz briefly until the pastry comes together into a ball of dough. Remove the pastry, wrap it in clingfilm (plastic wrap) and freeze for 10 minutes.

Plunge the asparagus into a pan of boiling water, lift out after a minute, drain and refresh under cold running water. Now, plunge the spinach leaves into the same boiling water for a minute, lift out, drain and refresh under cold running water.

Roll out the pastry on a floured board, lift it over the baking tray and carefully line it, cutting the edges with a sharp knife. Prick the pastry base with a fork, line with another sheet of baking parchment (wax paper) and some ceramic baking beans and bake blind for 10 minutes. Remove the paper and ceramic beans and bake for a further 5 minutes to cook the base a little more.

Cover the pastry base with the spinach leaves. Mix the crème fraîche and the hard cheese into the beaten eggs and season with a sprinkling of nutmeg, salt and pepper. Pour the mixture over the spinach, then arrange all the asparagus in a line from one end to the other. Sprinkle with cayenne pepper if desired and bake in the oven for about 30 minutes, or until the pastry is golden and the filling set.

Serve warm with a big mixed herb salad or leave to cool and then chill until needed.

Mushroom and Mozzarella Lasagne

If you use ripe vine tomatoes, the sauce should be light, sweet and full of flavour, which will contrast beautifully with the rich, deep, intense flavour of the mushrooms. You can go mad and use double or treble the amount of dried wild mushrooms, and you can use wild fresh mushrooms in place of the cultivated ones – pure magic! This recipe can be frozen.

Serves 6

GF   V

Tomato sauce

2 large onions, finely chopped

2 tablespoons cold pressed extra virgin olive oil

1.5kg/3½lbs fresh ripe vine or plum tomatoes, peeled, quartered and cores and seeds removed (to remove skins, submerge tomatoes in a bowl of boiling water, slash the skins and they will start to loosen. Remove with a sharp knife)

Sea salt and freshly ground black pepper

2 large garlic cloves, crushed

Minced chilli in oil (according to taste)

2 bay leaves

2 heaped teaspoons fresh thyme leaves

2 heaped tablespoons sun-dried tomato sauce

Mushroom filling

500g/1lb 2oz large, flat chestnut or portabella mushrooms

500g/1lb 2oz large, flat horse or field mushrooms

60g/2oz dried mixed wild mushrooms or your favourite kind

4 tablespoons cold pressed extra virgin olive oil

1 tablespoon fresh thyme leaves

1 large garlic clove, crushed

Sea salt and freshly ground black pepper

Sprinkling of freshly grated nutmeg

Lasagne
150g/6 sheets wheat-free* or Orgran rice and corn lasagne (see page 305 for stockist)
500g/2 cups organic ricotta cheese
255g/2 cups reduced-fat grated mozzarella cheese
Sprinkling of cayenne pepper

33cm/13in long and 20cm/8in wide ovenproof baking and serving dish

---

* coeliacs please use gluten-free ingredients

Preheat the oven to 180°C/350°F/Gas mark 4.

Make the tomato sauce first. Gently cook the onions over a low heat in the oil in a non-stick pan but do not brown them. Chop up the prepared tomatoes and once the onions are soft, stir the tomatoes into the onions along with all the remaining sauce ingredients. Simmer the sauce for 40 minutes, vigorously stirring with a wooden spoon from time to time until it is a soft pulp. Adjust the seasoning and then leave the sauce to cool.

Make the mushroom filling. Peel and trim the various cultivated fresh mushrooms, quarter them and slice them thinly. Sauté them with the dried wild mushrooms in a big non-stick pan in the oil, over a medium heat, until they have softened – about 10 minutes. Stir in the thyme and garlic and toss the mushrooms to ensure that they get evenly coated with oil and cooked through. Season the mushrooms with salt, pepper and grated nutmeg and leave to cool.

Spread a little less than half of the tomato sauce over the base of the baking dish. Cover the sauce with 3 strips of lasagne. You may have to break one piece and jiggle the pieces around to fit. Spoon the mushrooms all over the lasagne sheets, making sure that you take them right to the edges of the dish. Using a tablespoon, spoon the ricotta in blobs all over the mushrooms. Press the remaining 3 sheets of lasagne over the cheese. Again, you may have to break one piece up. Cover with the remaining tomato sauce, sprinkle with the mozzarella and dust with cayenne pepper. Bake in the oven for 45 minutes or until it is a dark golden colour, bubbling and an inserted knife goes through the soft lasagne sheets.

Fresh Pea Quiche

Quiche is still such a good way of filling up family or friends for lunches, weekend picnics and holidays. You can make double the quantity or make mini versions for parties. Mini cup muffin trays, available from all good cook shops, are excellent for this.

Serves 6   GF   V

Pastry
255g/2¼ cups wheat-free flour mix*
125g/4½oz organic butter, cut into 5 pieces
1 large organic free-range egg
Pinch of sea salt
A little cold water

Filling
1 tablespoon cold pressed extra virgin olive oil
1 onion, finely chopped
1 teaspoon herbes de Provence (mixed herbs can be used as an alternative)
400g/14oz fresh green peas in their pods, shelled
1 tablespoon fresh tarragon leaves
4 large organic free-range eggs, beaten in a bowl
Sea salt and freshly ground black pepper
Freshly grated nutmeg
255g/1 cup virtually fat-free fromage frais

Optional
30g/¼ cup freshly grated reduced-fat hard cheese and a sprinkling of cayenne pepper

ceramic baking beans
28cm/11in quiche dish or fluted loose-bottomed tart tin (pan)

* coeliacs please use gluten-free ingredients

Preheat the oven to 200°C/400°F/Gas mark 6.

Make the pastry by briefly blending all the ingredients, except the water, in a food processor until it resembles breadcrumbs. Add a little water and whizz briefly until the pastry comes together into a ball of dough. Remove the pastry, wrap it in clingfilm (plastic wrap) and freeze for 10 minutes.

Heat the oil in a non-stick frying pan (skillet) and cook the onions over a medium heat until soft but not brown. Cook the peas in boiling water until tender, drain and refresh under cold running water. Stir the herbes de Provence into the onions and cook for a few more minutes.

Roll out the pastry on a floured board into a large enough piece and gently lift it over the quiche dish. Line the dish with the pastry and even off the edges with a sharp knife. Prick the base with a fork in a few places, cover with a layer of non-stick baking parchment (wax paper), fill with a layer of ceramic baking beans and bake blind for 10 minutes. Remove the paper and beans, return to the oven and bake for another 5 minutes.

Put the warm onions into a bowl with the peas, tarragon, beaten eggs, salt, pepper and grated nutmeg and mix thoroughly. Stir in the fromage frais until the mixture is evenly combined. Pour the mixture into the pastry case. Sprinkle with cheese and cayenne if using, and bake in the oven for 20 minutes until the pastry is golden brown and the filling is just firm. Serve warm or cold with a selection of salads.

Broad Bean and Spinach Frittata

What a marvellous way to get the family to eat spinach and broad (fava) beans, heavily disguised in this clever Spanish dish.

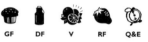

Serves 4–6

GF DF V RF Q&E

You need about 1kg/2¼lbs of broad (fava) beans in their pods to give you 400g/14oz of whole beans or 400g/14oz of frozen and defrosted broad (fava) beans
255g/10oz fresh spinach leaves, trimmed
6 organic free-range eggs
7g/¼oz chopped flat-leaf parsley
60g/¾ cup freshly grated pecorino cheese or dairy-free cheese (see page 305 for stockist)
30g/2 tablespoons organic butter or dairy-free margarine
Sea salt and freshly ground black pepper

25.5cm/10in heavy-based, non-stick frying pan (skillet)

Cook the fresh or defrosted broad (fava) beans in boiling water until just tender, drain and refresh under cold running water. Pop the broad (fava) beans out of their skins and discard the skins.

Meanwhile, blanch the spinach in a big pan of boiling water for about 2 minutes, drain and refresh it under cold running water. Gently squeeze the excess water out of the spinach and then lay it out on thick sheets of absorbent kitchen paper to soak up any remaining moisture.

Beat the eggs lightly with a fork in a big bowl. Stir in the broad (fava) beans, spinach, parsley, three-quarters of the cheese and season with salt and pepper. Melt the margarine or butter in the pan until foaming, pour in the egg mixture and turn the heat down as low as possible.

When the eggs are on the verge of setting, preheat the grill (broiler). Sprinkle the remaining cheese over the frittata, slide the pan under the grill (broiler) and cook until golden. Transfer the frittata to a clean board, leave it to cool then cut into 4–6 wedges.

Vegetables and
Accompaniments ...

Katie's Parsnips

My sister-in-law Katie provided this recipe. These delicious parsnips liven up roast chicken, pheasant, game or meat. Don't be tempted to use old, out-of-date spices – using fresh spices really makes a difference to the taste of any dish.

Serves 6

GF   DF   V

1 heaped teaspoon cumin seeds
1 heaped teaspoon ground coriander
½ teaspoon turmeric powder
A pinch of cayenne
Sea salt and freshly ground black pepper
200ml/¾ cup coconut cream or creamed coconut
2 tablespoons cold pressed extra virgin olive oil
1kg/2¼lb trimmed parsnips, peeled and cut into halves or quarters if large

Preheat the oven to 200°C/400°F/Gas mark 6.

In a bowl, mix all the spices and seasoning with the coconut cream and oil.

Cook the parsnips in boiling water until softened. Drain and refresh them under cold running water then set them aside for 5 minutes in the colander. Put the parsnips in a roasting dish large enough to allow them to lie in a single layer. Pour the spice mixture over the parsnips and toss until they are well coated.

Roast the parsnips for about 1 hour until they are golden and crispy on both sides. Serve immediately so that they remain crispy.

Cauliflower with Breadcrumbs

I love those seasonal big gleaming white cauliflowers, not the trendy miniatures you can buy all year round in the supermarket. Cauliflower is delicious covered in parsley sauce and served with roast meats, and I often add cauliflower to macaroni cheese, but now that I make fresh wheat-free bread every day this has become my favourite recipe.

Serves 6

GF   DF   V   Q&E

100g/3½oz organic butter or dairy-free margarine

115g/4oz fresh wheat-free breadcrumbs* (not too fine)

1 garlic clove, crushed

Finely grated rind of 1 unwaxed lemon

2 heaped tablespoons chopped fresh parsley

Sea salt and freshly ground black pepper

1 large cauliflower, separated into even-sized florets

* coeliacs please use gluten-free ingredients

Melt 55g/2oz of the butter or margarine in a non-stick frying pan (skillet) and once it is foaming stir in the breadcrumbs. Fry the crumbs until golden and crisp, then stir in the garlic, finely grated lemon rind and parsley. Season the crumbs with salt and pepper and set aside.

Steam the cauliflower for about 5 minutes until just soft then sauté the florets in another pan with the remaining butter or margarine until tinged with golden brown.

Transfer the cauliflower to a warm serving dish, sprinkle with the crumbs and serve.

Creamy Bread Sauce

This traditional British sauce is served not only with roast chicken or turkey but also with game birds such as partridge, woodcock and grouse. The sauce contrasts well with cranberry sauce, which is also often served alongside Christmas turkey and game birds.

Serves 8

GF   DF   V

1 onion, quartered and studded with 4 cloves

2 bay leaves, plus extra to garnish

500ml/2 cups organic milk or dairy-free soya milk

170g/6oz fresh white wheat-free bread (crusts removed), made into crumbs (see page 304 for stockist)

Plenty of freshly grated nutmeg

55g/2oz organic butter or dairy-free margarine

Up to 125ml/½ cup organic double cream, Elmlea double cream (a blend of buttermilk and vegetable oils) or Provamel dairy-free Soya Dream (see page 304 for stockist)

Sea salt and freshly ground black pepper

Put the onion, bay leaves and milk into a non-stick pan. Heat gently on low heat for about 15 minutes, stirring occasionally. Remove the onion and bay leaves and add the breadcrumbs, nutmeg, butter or margarine. Heat gently for about 5 minutes and stir in enough cream to give a nice thick consistency – amount needed will depend on the absorbency of the bread used. Season with a little salt and pepper and serve.

Cranberry and Pistachio Rice

This rather exotic rice dish is delicious with roast or sautéed game birds, rich dark meat or game casseroles. I have also used it as an accompaniment to poached chicken breasts with a light creamy sauce.

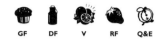

Serves 6–8

340g/12oz basmati rice
A pinch of saffron strands
100g/3½oz packet dried cranberries
55g/½ cup shelled pistachios, coarsely chopped
Sea salt and freshly ground black pepper

Rinse the rice several times, tip into a pan and cover with water. Bring the rice to the boil, reduce the heat slightly and stir in the saffron, cranberries and plenty of salt and pepper.

Cook until the rice is tender and the water has been absorbed. Spoon the rice into a serving dish and scatter the pistachio nuts over the top.

Crispy Courgettes with Breadcrumbs

This is another delicious Italian recipe that can easily be made now that there are so many good wheat-free breads around. You can parboil the courgettes (zucchini) and make the crumbs a few hours in advance and put the dish together at the last minute.

Serves 4   GF   DF   V   Q&E

750g/4 large courgettes (zucchini), trimmed and cut into diagonal slices

Topping
85g/3oz organic butter or dairy-free margarine
100g/3½oz fresh wheat-free breadcrumbs*
1 large garlic clove, finely chopped
Finely grated rind of 1 unwaxed lemon
2 tablespoons chopped fresh parsley

* coeliacs please use gluten-free ingredients

Cook the courgettes (zucchini) in boiling water for a few minutes until softened. Drain and refresh them under cold running water.

Meanwhile, melt 55g/2oz of the butter or margarine in a non-stick frying pan (skillet). As soon as it is foaming, add the crumbs and fry over moderate heat until crisp and golden. Stir in the garlic and transfer the crumbs to a warm plate.

Heat the rest of the butter or margarine in the pan and sauté the courgettes (zucchini) until tinged with gold. Return the crumbs to the pan, add the grated lemon rind and parsley and sauté for a few minutes. Serve in a warm dish to accompany roast poultry, game, meat or fish.

Sage and Hazelnut Stuffing

Here is a wheat-free stuffing for your Christmas or Easter turkey. It is enough to stuff a 4.5–5.4kg/10–12lb bird. If you are cooking a smaller bird, keep any excess stuffing and mould it into balls that you can roast with the potatoes. Use your favourite recipe for cooking your turkey exactly the way you like it. I roast my turkey wrapped in plenty of bacon to keep it moist and lightly cover it with mixed herbs and freshly ground black pepper. To protect the bird I lightly wrap it in oiled foil but remove this about 45 minutes before the end of the cooking time in order to brown the turkey breast. I set the turkey in a big roasting dish with water, stock, white wine, onion, bay leaves and sliced carrot, which makes the most delicious gravy. I thicken the gravy with pure cornflour (cornstarch) and serve the turkey with traditional Creamy Bread Sauce (see page 190). Note that you need to soak the dried fruit the day before you make the remainder of the recipe.

Stuffs 2 chickens or 1 turkey   **GF**   **DF**   **V**   **Q&E**

100g/⅔ cup raisins, soaked overnight in 60ml/¼ cup sherry

340g/12oz red onion, very thinly chopped in a food processor

55g/2oz organic butter or dairy-free margarine

1 tablespoon unrefined golden caster (superfine) sugar

Finely grated rind and juice of 1 unwaxed orange

2 heaped tablespoons chopped fresh sage

100g/3½oz packet chopped toasted hazelnuts

100g/3½oz gluten-free white breadcrumbs (see page 305 for stockist)

Sea salt, freshly ground black pepper and freshly grated nutmeg

1 large organic free-range egg, beaten

455g/1lb gluten-free sausage meat (see page 306 for stockist or use skinned sausages if they are easier to find)

Fry the onions gently in the butter or margarine until golden and then add the sugar and orange rind and juice. Continue cooking until the onions are soft and sticky. Stir in the sage, hazelnuts, breadcrumbs and plenty of seasoning and beat in the egg. Mix the sausage meat in using a wooden spoon and then stir in the raisins along with the sherry.

Adjust the seasoning if necessary and the stuffing is ready for use.

Parmesan and Olive Oil Mash

This simple Italian-style potato dish is delicious served with roast chicken or other roast meats. I think that the flavours are too strong to serve with fish but you can certainly serve it with vegetarian dishes.

Serves 4

GF   DF   V   Q&E

900g/2lb boiling potatoes, peeled and cut into quarters

Sea salt and freshly ground black pepper

55g/2oz organic butter or dairy-free margarine

2 tablespoons cold pressed extra virgin olive oil

30g/1oz grated fresh Parmesan or dairy-free Florentino Parmazano (see page 306 for stockist)

A pinch of freshly grated nutmeg

Boil the potatoes in a pan of water until cooked through. Drain and return to the pan. Mash the potatoes until light and fluffy, stir in the remaining ingredients and adjust the seasoning.

Serve straight away or keep covered and warm until needed.

Leeks Napolitano

In the grim days of February, I remind my parents how satisfying it is for them to battle against the bitter, freezing north Norfolk wind, and venture down to the kitchen garden, to dig up a bundle of sturdy leeks for our lunch! Very conveniently, I cannot possibly dig them up myself, with such a bad back, but I can cook a delicious lunch using them!

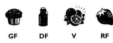

Serves 3   GF   DF   V   RF

---

1 onion, finely chopped
1 teaspoon dried thyme leaves
1 teaspoon dried herbes de Provence (mixed herbs can be used as an alternative)
1 tablespoon cold pressed extra virgin olive oil plus extra for sprinkling
400g/14oz can chopped tomatoes
1 teaspoon allergy-free vegetable bouillon powder
Sea salt and freshly ground black pepper
7g/¼oz flat-leaf parsley, finely chopped
500g/1lb 2oz prepared leeks
Sprinkling of cayenne pepper

Preheat the oven to 180°C/350°F/Gas mark 4.

Cook the onion and herbs in a pan with the tablespoon of oil until nearly soft but not browned. Stir in the tomatoes, bouillon powder and pepper. Simmer for another 20 minutes or until completely soft. Remove from the heat and stir in the parsley.

Cut each leek into 3 pieces and plunge into a pan of boiling water to cook for 5 minutes. Drain and refresh under cold water. Transfer the leeks to an ovenproof serving dish, arranging them neatly.

Spoon the tomato sauce all over the leeks and sprinkle with a little oil and cayenne pepper. Bake in the oven for about 25 minutes until the leeks are soft.

Coleslaw

Ready-made coleslaw is much maligned, but the homemade version is always delicious. Coleslaw is perfect for munching with a baked potato for winter lunches and delicious with new potatoes in their skins in summer.

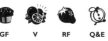

Serves 4 with baked potatoes or 6 as part of a picnic

GF   V   RF   Q&E

½ a small firm white cabbage (400g/14oz), halved and very finely sliced
300g/11oz organic carrots, coarsely grated
1 tablespoon freshly pressed bottled apple juice
5 heaped tablespoons virtually fat-free fromage frais
110g/¾ cup shelled Brazil nuts, coarsely chopped
Sea salt and freshly ground black pepper
30g/¼ cup sesame seeds
15g/½oz finely chopped parsley leaves

Optional
Dash Worcestershire sauce* and Tabasco*

* coeliacs please use gluten-free ingredients

Put the sliced cabbage and grated carrots into a big salad bowl. In a small bowl, mix the apple juice and fromage frais together and then combine with the cabbage.

Mix in the nuts, salt, pepper, Worcestershire and Tabasco sauces. Sprinkle with the sesame seeds and parsley. Cover and chill the coleslaw until needed but eat it on the day of making.

The Big Book of Wheat-Free Cooking

Barbecued Vegetables with Dipping Sauce

The art of the successful barbecue is advance planning. Prepare and pre-cook everything you possibly can and keep it chilled until needed. This way you will have time to enjoy the party too! Do not be tempted to keep seafood, chicken or meat languishing around in the sunshine or near the heat of the fire, or there could be a number of upset tummies around.

Here are five easy recipes that all the family can enjoy. Each one will serve eight people. Decorate all the plates of cooked foods with sprigs of fresh rosemary or other herbs. You can easily add king prawns (jumbo shrimp) and chicken breasts to the barbecue. If so, then make up some more of the marinade for the spicy squash quarters and brush it over the prawns (shrimp) or chicken.

Red Onions with Rosemary Dressing

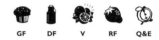

GF   DF   V   RF   Q&E

3 large red onions, cut into 8 wedges

3 tablespoons cold pressed extra virgin olive oil plus a little extra for brushing

Sea salt and freshly ground black pepper

Cayenne pepper

2 tablespoons balsamic vinegar

3 teaspoons chopped fresh rosemary

8 bamboo skewers, soaked in warm water for 5 minutes

Thread the onion wedges on to the bamboo skewers. Brush both sides with the oil, season with salt, pepper and a light sprinkling of cayenne.

Barbecue the onion kebabs for 30–35 minutes, turning from time to time and brushing with extra oil when necessary until tender and lightly charred.

To make the dressing, mix together the balsamic vinegar, the 3 tablespoons of olive oil and the chopped rosemary. Drizzle over the cooked onions and serve.

Sweet Potato Wedges

You can speed up this recipe by parboiling the potatoes. It is a good idea to add a little lemon juice to the water to prevent discolouration. Refresh the semi-cooked potatoes under cold running water, leave them in cold water and keep covered until needed.

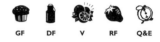

GF   DF   V   RF   Q&E

900g/2lb medium-sized sweet potatoes, peeled and halved
Juice of ½ a small lemon (if parboiling)
2 large garlic cloves, crushed
4 tablespoons cold pressed extra virgin olive oil
3 teaspoons finely chopped sage
Sea salt and freshly ground black pepper
1 teaspoon ground paprika

8 bamboo skewers, soaked in warm water for 5 minutes

Parboil the potatoes in boiling water with the lemon juice for 10 minutes. Drain and refresh as suggested above.

When you are ready to barbecue, slice the potatoes into thick wedges. Divide the wedges into 8 portions. Push them along each skewer, keeping them close together but not touching.

Combine the crushed garlic and olive oil with the sage, seasoning and paprika, and brush it all over the potatoes. Cook over medium–hot coals for 20–30 minutes until tender and lightly browned. Serve with the dipping sauce on page 200.

Spicy Squash Quarters

Apply the same parboiling technique to these squash quarters as for the Sweet Potato Wedges until they are just soft.

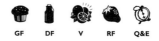

GF	DF	V	RF	Q&E

2 small butternut squash, quartered and seeded

Marinade
2 tablespoons cold pressed extra virgin olive oil
Sea salt and freshly ground black pepper
2 large garlic cloves, crushed
2 teaspoons ground cumin
2 teaspoons ground coriander
Sprinkling of cayenne pepper

Mix all the marinade ingredients together in a bowl and brush them over the parboiled but cooled squash quarters. Cook over medium-hot coals for 20–30 minutes until tender, turning occasionally. Serve with the dipping sauce on page 200.

Charred Courgettes

You could also use aubergines (eggplants) but I am so allergic to them that I cannot even touch them without coming out in a rash and definitely couldn't test the recipe for you, so I am afraid I will have to leave that one to you!

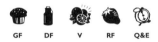

4 large courgettes (zucchini), halved lengthways
Cold pressed extra virgin olive oil
I large garlic clove, crushed
2 teaspoons finely chopped fresh rosemary
Sea salt and freshly ground black pepper

Score a crisscross pattern on the fleshy side of the courgettes (zucchini). Brush lightly with olive oil and sprinkle with the remaining ingredients.

Cook the courgettes (zucchini) for 10 minutes, or until just tender, over medium–hot coals, turning occasionally until the courgettes (zucchini) are slightly charred at the edges. Serve with the dipping sauce on page 200.

Dipping Sauce

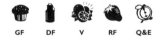

2 tablespoons clear honey
I tablespoon whole-grain mustard*
I tablespoon lemon juice
4 tablespoons soy sauce*
8 tablespoons tomato ketchup
Chilli sauce*, minced chilli in oil or chopped fresh chillies, according to taste
Sea salt and freshly ground black pepper

* coeliacs please use gluten-free ingredients

To make the dipping sauce, simply combine all the ingredients, then transfer to a serving bowl and serve with the barbecued vegetables.

The Big Book of Wheat-Free Cooking

Cold Desserts ...

Peach and Amaretti Tart

Peaches combined with amaretti have long been a traditional Italian partnership. Here I have put them into a tart to make a more substantial pudding. It's delicious served with dairy or dairy-free vanilla ice cream or crème fraîche.

GF   DF   V

Serves 8

Pastry

225g/2 cups wheat-free flour mix*
115g/4oz organic butter or dairy-free margarine
1 organic free-range egg
A little chilled filtered water

Filling

200g/7oz organic butter or dairy-free margarine
85g/scant ½ cup unrefined golden caster (superfine) sugar
100g/3½oz amaretti biscuits* (almond macaroons), crushed – check the label to ensure that they are gluten free
155g/5½oz Doves Farm organic Lemon Zest Cookies or other gluten-free brands, crushed
115g/4oz ground almonds
4 organic free-range eggs
1 tablespoon lemon juice
6 ripe peaches, peeled, halved and stones discarded (if the skins don't come off easily, stand the peaches in a bowl of boiling water, score the skin lightly with a knife and leave for a few minutes)

25.5cm/10in fluted non-stick flan tin (pan) lined with a circle of non-stick baking parchment (wax paper) or Bake-O-Glide

* coeliacs please use gluten-free ingredients

The Big Book of Wheat-Free Cooking

Preheat the oven to 180°C/350°F/Gas mark 4.

Make the pastry first. Put the flour and butter or margarine in a food processor and combine briefly until they resemble breadcrumbs. Add the egg and blend again until a smooth dough forms. You may need to add some water depending on the absorbency of the flour. Remove the dough, wrap in clingfilm (plastic wrap) and chill for half an hour.

Meanwhile, put the butter, sugar, crushed amaretti (almond macaroons), lemon zest cookies and almonds into a food processor and whiz until it blends together. Add the eggs and lemon juice and process into a coarse paste; scrape the bowl with a spatula and process briefly again.

Roll out the pastry on a floured surface to fit the prepared flan tin (pan). Line the tin (pan) with the pastry and trim the edges. Spread the mixture over the base of the pastry case; arrange the peaches over the top, pressing them gently into the mixture.

Bake in the oven for about 55 minutes until golden brown and firm to the touch. Cool the tart in the tin (pan) before removing to a serving plate.

Cranberry Trifle

Cranberries make an excellent seasonal change from the raspberry and banana combination that is so traditional in Christmas trifles. The key to cooking cranberries successfully is to simmer them with a little bit of water until they soften and pop, then add the sugar – any earlier and the skins will toughen.

OPTIONAL

Serves 12

GF   DF   V

Custard

810ml/3¼ cups full fat organic milk or Provamel organic vanilla soya milk

1 vanilla pod, split lengthways

115g/generous ½ cup unrefined golden caster (superfine) sugar

6 organic free-range egg yolks

2 tablespoons pure cornflour (cornstarch), dissolved in a little cold filtered water

250ml/1 cup chilled organic double cream or Provamel dairy-free Soya Dream

Trifle

225g/8oz fresh or frozen cranberries

55g/⅓ cup unrefined golden caster (superfine) sugar

Finely grated rind and the juice of 1 unwaxed orange

2 teaspoons ground arrowroot, dissolved in a little cold filtered water

16 slices of The Village Bakery organic wheat-free lemon cake* (see page 304 for stockist) – those on a
   gluten- or dairy-free diet should use an alternative cake

Any kind of orange-based liqueur* or some fresh orange juice

8 amaretti morbidi or other almond macaroons (check label for wheat- or gluten-free)

40g/½ cup flaked almonds, toasted until golden under the grill (broiler)

Optional for dairy recipe only

500ml/2 cups of organic double (heavy) cream, whipped for the topping

* coeliacs please use gluten-free ingredients

Make the custard first. Put the milk, vanilla pod and half the sugar in a non-stick pan. Place the pan over a low heat and cook until it reaches boiling point, stirring occasionally. Remove from the heat and take out the vanilla pod.

Beat the egg yolks, the remaining sugar and the dissolved cornflour (cornstarch) in a food processor until pale then, with the machine still running, pour in the hot milk and blend briefly until smooth. Return the custard to the pan and cook over low heat, stirring all the time, until the custard is very thick and at boiling point but do not let it boil or it may curdle.

Pour the custard through a sieve into a bowl, immediately stir in the cream or Soya Dream and leave to cool, stirring from time to time. Cover with clingfilm (plastic wrap) and chill in the refrigerator until needed.

Put the cranberries, sugar and finely grated orange rind and juice in a pan and simmer until the cranberries are soft. Stir in the dissolved arrowroot, cook until thick and leave to cool.

Cover the base and the sides of a large, glass serving bowl with the slices of lemon cake. Sprinkle with liqueur or some fresh orange juice if preferred. Spoon half the custard into the bowl, spreading it all over the sponge. Spoon in all the cranberries and spread them around. Scatter the crumbled amaretti (almond macaroons) all over the cranberries then spoon over the remaining custard and sprinkle it with flaked almonds. Cover and chill until needed.

If you can eat dairy products you can spread whipped cream over the final layer of custard and then decorate with the flaked almonds.

Chestnut Parfait with Chocolate Sauce

This wonderfully rich pudding can be made weeks in advance and taken out of the deep-freeze about 20 minutes before serving. Puddings like this are always a great help, as they leave you more time to relax with your guests.

Serves 6–8

GF   V

55g/⅓ cup large sultanas (golden raisins), soaked in boiling water for 15 minutes, drained and macerated in 4 tablespoons of good quality brandy or rum overnight

Ice cream
4 large organic free-range egg yolks

130g/⅔ cup unrefined golden caster (superfine) sugar

255g/9oz can sweetened chestnut purée (Merchant Gourmet) or if unavailable use 255g/9oz unsweetened chestnut purée

90g/¼ cup golden (corn) syrup

375ml/¼ cups organic double (heavy) cream

Chocolate sauce
150g/5½ × 1oz squares dark chocolate (73% pure cocoa)

30g/1oz organic butter

125ml/½ cup full fat organic milk

1kg/2¼lb loaf tin (pan), lightly oiled and lined with clingfilm (plastic wrap)

Using an electric whisk, beat the egg yolks in a heatproof bowl until smooth and pale then set them aside. Tip the sugar into a pan, add 5 tablespoons of filtered water and slowly dissolve over low heat. When the mixture is clear, increase the heat, bring to the boil and cook for 6 minutes. Immediately pour the sugar syrup into the eggs, whisking steadily as you pour. Continue to whisk for 4 minutes and then leave the mixture to cool.

In another bowl, beat the chestnut purée with the golden (corn) syrup, if using, then mix in the brandy- or rum-soaked sultanas (golden raisins) and all the liquid. Whisk the cream into soft peaks in a separate bowl then combine it with the chestnut mixture and finally with the egg mixture.

Spoon the mixture into the tin (pan) and smooth over the surface. Wrap in clingfilm (plastic wrap) and freeze until needed or until solid.

Take the parfait out of the deep-freeze 20 minutes before it is needed. Meanwhile, make the chocolate sauce. Put the chocolate and butter in a heatproof bowl over a pan of simmering water and stir until it is melted, smooth and glossy. Gradually stir in the milk until the sauce reaches pouring consistency.

Unwrap the parfait and turn it out onto a flat plate. Cut the parfait into 6–8 slices and place each one in the centre of a plate. Drizzle with the warm chocolate sauce and serve immediately.

Super Cheat's Orange Creams

If you keep all the ingredients in the refrigerator, you can put this ultra easy dessert together in minutes just before serving. Choose smallish wine glasses so that the cream doesn't look mean and serve with a pile of pretty paper-wrapped (wheat-free) amaretti* for no cooking at all!

GF   V   Q&E

Serves 6

325g/11½oz jar luxury orange curd*
750g/3 cups half-fat crème fraîche
Finely grated rind of ½ an unwaxed orange plus a little extra for decoration
8 amaretti morbidi (soft almond macaroons) or other wheat-free brands*, broken into quarters

---

* coeliacs please use gluten-free ingredients

Place the first three ingredients in a mixing bowl in the given order and mix them together using a metal spoon. Fold in the amaretti pieces (almond macaroons) and spoon the mixture into six wine glasses. Decorate with a tiny sprinkling of finely grated orange rind, cover and chill or serve.

Caramel and Chocolate Sundaes

There are moments when an instant sweet treat is needed and this is my stand-by pudding when I haven't had time to drive to the shops. The Provamel desserts are long life so I keep them in the cold larder or the refrigerator. I always have amaretti biscuits, bananas and dark chocolate lurking around my kitchen so it doesn't take long to put the whole lot together!

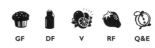

GF   DF   V   RF   Q&E

Serves 2

2 Provamel chocolate-flavoured dairy-free desserts
1 medium ripe banana, thinly sliced
2 Provamel caramel-flavoured dairy-free desserts
4 amaretti morbidi (wheat-free soft almond macaroons)*, coarsely crumbled
15g/½ × 1oz square coarsely grated dark dairy-free chocolate* (73% pure cocoa)

* coeliacs please use gluten-free ingredients

Choose two large wine glasses. Begin by putting a layer of chocolate dessert in the bottom of each glass. Level this off and cover with a layer of banana slices.

In a small bowl, mix the caramel dessert with half the amaretti (almond macaroons) and then cover the bananas with this mixture. Decorate with the remaining crumbled amaretti (almond macaroons) and a thick layer of grated chocolate and serve immediately.

Pine Nut Semifreddo

Semifreddo literally means 'half cold' therefore this isn't quite an ice cream. You can make it a few days in advance and freeze until needed. Take it out of the deep-freeze to soften about 10 minutes before serving. Serve the semifreddo with hot roast fruit such as peaches or cherries. Roasted fresh pineapple or plums in winter are also delicious.

Serves 8

GF   V

Praline

200g/1cup unrefined golden caster (superfine) sugar

4 tablespoons filtered water

100g/3½oz packet pine nuts, grilled (broiled) or baked until golden

Semifreddo

1 vanilla pod

4 large organic free-range eggs, separated

4 tablespoons unrefined golden caster (superfine) sugar

310ml/1¼ cups organic double (heavy) cream

A pinch of fine salt

Optional

Roast seasonal fruits, chocolate sauce or seasonal fruit purée to serve

Make the praline first. Put the sugar and water into a pan and heat gently until it starts to bubble. Shake the pan from time to time until the sugar syrup is clear and then turns into a dark caramel. Immediately remove the pan from the heat. Tip the pan away from you and pour in the pine nuts.

Carefully pour the caramel over a lightly oiled baking tray and leave until cold and set. Break up the praline once it has set, put it in a plastic bag, seal and bash with a rolling pin until it becomes a coarse powder. Leave to one side.

Make the semifreddo mixture. Halve the vanilla pod and, using a teaspoon, scrape out the seeds into a bowl containing the egg yolks and sugar. Whisk the mixture until very pale and creamy.

In a separate bowl, whisk the cream into soft peaks and, in another bowl, whisk the egg whites with a pinch of salt into firm and stiff peaks.

Fold the cream into the egg yolk mixture then fold in the egg whites and the crushed praline. Line a standard-sized bread tin (pan) with enough clingfilm (plastic wrap) to overlap the edges. Spoon the mixture into the tin (pan), cover with the clingfilm (plastic wrap) and freeze for at least 4 hours or until firm.

Turn out the semifreddo, remove the clingfilm (plastic wrap), cut into slices and decorate according to season.

Honey, Almond and Thyme Ice Cream

Use a flower or herb honey for a deep rich flavour – orange blossom is particularly good in this recipe.
I always make double the quantity so that I have enough to set aside for an impromptu pudding.

Serves 4

GF **V**

310ml/1¼ cups organic milk

4 large organic free-range egg yolks

125ml/½ cup high quality honey

½ teaspoon thyme oil (see page 306 for stockist) or use 4 sprigs of fresh thyme heated in the milk and
    discarded before processing

310ml/1¼ cups organic double (heavy) cream

55g/½ cup flaked almonds, toasted until golden brown

Heat the milk in a non-stick pan, over medium heat, until it reaches boiling point then remove from the heat. Meanwhile, beat the egg yolks, honey and ½ teaspoon of thyme oil together in a food processor until smooth. Gradually pour the hot milk through the funnel, blending all the time until you have a thin custard.

Scrape the custard into the pan and cook gently, over low heat, until the custard thickens. Do not boil the custard or it will separate. Add a few more drops of thyme oil if you prefer a stronger flavour but be careful it doesn't become overpowering. Leave the thickened custard to cool in a bowl.

Gently fold the cream and almonds into the cold custard and transfer to a prepared ice cream maker. Churn until softly frozen and serve with baked fruits.

Alternatively, transfer to a container, seal and freeze until needed.

Brown Bread Ice Cream

This ice cream is ultra quick and easy; it's really just whipped cream and caramelized breadcrumbs. You need to serve it with a fruit coulis or sauce. You can use any soft summer berries in summer, damsons in autumn (fall) or dried apricots in winter.

GF   V

Serves 4

115g/4oz light wheat-free brown bread* crusts removed (see page 304 for stockist)
55g/⅓ cup unrefined soft brown sugar
2 large organic free-range egg whites
310ml/1¼ cups organic double (heavy) cream

Optional
287g/10oz jar fruit coulis or make your own seasonal fruit purée

4 large ramekins or large individual tin pudding basins lined with clingfilm (plastic wrap)

* coeliacs please use gluten-free ingredients

Make the bread into breadcrumbs using a food processor. Add the sugar to the food processor and mix in briefly. Preheat the grill (broiler) until hot and line the grill (broiler) pan with a layer of oiled foil.

Sprinkle the breadcrumbs over the foil and toast them until golden, then break them up and toast on the other side. Don't burn them or they will taste horrible. Transfer the crumbs to a baking sheet and leave to cool.

Whisk the egg whites to stiff peaks in a bowl. In a separate bowl, whisk the cream until thick. Fold the cold breadcrumbs into the cream and then gently fold in the egg whites. Spoon the mixture into the prepared ramekins or pudding basins, cover with clingfilm (plastic wrap) and freeze until needed.

Remove the clingfilm (plastic wrap), turn the ice creams out of the ramekins onto plates and serve drizzled with fruit coulis.

Please note that this recipe contains raw eggs.

Marmalade Ice Cream

Marmalade ice cream is not only delicious on its own but also with poached winter fruits or the Christmas Mincemeat Torte on page 251.

Serves 8–12

GF   V

225g/8oz fine shred mild-flavoured marmalade

2 tablespoons Cointreau

2 teaspoons glucose syrup

625ml/2½ cups organic milk

7 organic egg yolks

115g/½ cup vanilla caster (superfine) sugar (or unrefined golden caster sugar infused with vanilla seeds for a few days)

Finely grated rind of 1 unwaxed orange

560ml/2¼ cups organic double (heavy) cream, whipped into soft peaks

In a large bowl, mix the marmalade, Cointreau and glucose syrup. Heat the milk in a pan, over moderate heat, until it reaches boiling point. Meanwhile, blend the egg yolks and sugar in a food processor until smooth. Keep the food processor running while you quickly pour in the hot milk.

Transfer the custard to the milk pan and cook over low heat, stirring most of the time, until the custard reaches boiling point and has thickened considerably. Immediately combine the custard with the marmalade mixture and the grated orange rind. Stir occasionally to prevent a skin forming whilst the custard cools.

When the custard is cold, fold in the whipped cream and transfer to a prepared ice cream maker. You may need to make two batches. Churn the ice cream until softly frozen, scrape the mixture into a storage container, seal and freeze until needed.

Let the ice cream thaw for 10 minutes before serving.

Muscovado Meringues with Lime Cream

This is a perfect pudding for the summer, when you don't want to be in the kitchen. Meringues are very quick to make and can then be left for 4 hours whilst you enjoy the sunshine.

Serves 6 or 12

GF   V

6 organic free-range egg whites
340g/12oz unrefined light muscovado sugar, sieved
500ml/2 cups organic double (heavy) cream
Finely grated rind of 2 unwaxed limes

To serve

Slices of fresh ripe seasonal fruits (mango, pineapple, strawberry, raspberry, peaches or nectarines are all delicious), or frozen berry mixtures, defrosted

Preheat the oven to 130°C/250°F/Gas mark 1.

Whisk the egg whites in a large, clean and dry bowl until they form stiff peaks. Very gradually mix in the sugar, about a tablespoon at a time, whisking the mixture well each time so that the sugar dissolves and combines with the egg whites. Spoon the mixture onto lined baking sheets to form about 12 meringues and bake for about 4 hours until they are dry and hard. Cool and store until needed.

No more than a couple of hours before serving, whip the cream into soft peaks with the grated lime rind.

To serve 6: Take a pair of meringues, fill them with a large dollop of cream and squish them together. Place the meringues at a jaunty angle on each plate and serve with slices of fresh seasonal fruit.

To serve 12: Arrange the fruit on each plate, place a strategic dollop of lime cream on top and put a meringue jauntily across the top.

For a buffet party you can pile the meringues high on a big dish and decorate with fresh mint leaves and ripe berries.

Blackberry Meringue Chill

This quick and easy pudding can be made a few weeks in advance and frozen until about 1 hour before serving. It's a convenient way of using up any blackberries you may have left over after making the Blackberry and Apple Tarts on page 232.

GF   V

Serves 10

625ml/2½ cups organic double (heavy) cream
55g/⅓ cup unrefined light muscovado (soft brown) sugar
2 tablespoons cocoa powder or very finely grated dark chocolate
680g/1lb 8oz ripe blackberries
6 meringue nests, broken into small pieces
A little sieved unrefined icing (confectioners') sugar to decorate

2cm/8in round or square non-stick cake tin (pan) lined with clingfilm (plastic wrap)

Whip the cream until it holds its shape. Stir in the sugar and sift in the cocoa or chocolate.

Lightly mash 455g/1lb of the blackberries with a fork and fold into the cream along with the meringue pieces. Spoon the mixture into the prepared tin (pan). Smooth the top, cover and freeze for 4 hours or overnight.

Transfer the blackberry meringue chill into the refrigerator 1 hour before serving. Turn out onto a serving plate and scatter the remaining blackberries on top. Dust with icing (confectioners') sugar and serve.

Key Lime Pie

Key lime pie is a traditional recipe from Florida, where Key limes are grown. Key limes have a short season but other varieties of limes work just as well. Use unwaxed limes for the best flavour.

Serves 6–8

GF   V   Q&E

Base
250g/9oz Doves Farm organic gluten-free Lemon Zest Cookies
100g/3½oz organic butter

Filling
4 large organic free-range egg yolks
1 heaped tablespoon finely grated lime rind (use unwaxed limes)
400g/14oz can condensed milk
200ml/¾ cup fresh lime juice (4–5 limes) or slightly less if you don't want it to be too zesty

Optional
Crème fraîche to serve

24cm/9½in fluted, non-stick, loose-bottomed flan tin (pan)

Preheat the oven to 180°C/350°F/Gas mark 4.

Crush the cookies in a food processor until they resemble breadcrumbs. Melt the butter in a pan, remove from the heat and mix the crumbs and butter together in the pan. Spoon the mixture over the base of the prepared tin (pan) and press down evenly so that you have a smooth surface. Bake in the oven for about 10 minutes until crisp and golden.

Meanwhile, make the filling. Place the egg yolks and lime zest in a bowl and beat with an electric whisk for about 2 minutes until thickened slightly. Add the condensed milk, beat for a further 4 minutes before adding the lime juice and giving it a final quick whisk. Pour the mixture onto the baked crust and bake for 20 minutes or until it feels just set. Cool and then cover and chill until needed. Transfer the pie to a large plate and serve.

Lemon Cheesecake

I despaired of ever eating a cheesecake again until I came across the Tofutti range of cream cheeses and sour cream. I can now make all sorts of cheesecakes, as well as delicious dips and mousses.

GF   DF   V

Serves 8

Base

2 x 150g/5½oz packets Doves Farm organic gluten-free Lemon Zest Cookies

85g/3oz organic butter or dairy-free margarine

85g/scant ½ cup unrefined demerara sugar

Cheesecake

2 x 340g/12oz tubs dairy-free Tofutti Sour Supreme sour cream substitute (see page 305 for stockist)

Juice and finely grated lemon rind from 1 large unwaxed lemon

3 tablespoons unrefined golden caster (superfine) sugar

11.7g sachet/1 tablespoon gelatine powder dissolved in 150ml/generous ½ cup boiling filtered water or a vegetarian equivalent such as agar-agar

2 organic free-range egg whites, stiffly beaten

Finely grated rind of 1 unwaxed lemon for decoration

23cm/9in spring-form, loose-bottomed, non-stick cake tin (pan), lined with non-stick baking parchment (wax paper) or Bake-O-Glide

Preheat the oven to 180°C/350°F/Gas mark 4.

Make the base first. Break up the cookies and process them in a food processor until they resemble coarse breadcrumbs. In a small pan, heat the butter or margarine and sugar until melted, pour into the cookie crumbs and mix thoroughly. Press the crumb mixture into the lined tin (pan) and press down until it is flat and even.

Bake the cookie base in the oven for about 15 minutes; remove from the oven and leave to cool.

When the base is cold, make the filling. Place the cream or cream substitute, lemon juice and rind and sugar in a bowl and blend until very creamy. Stir in the dissolved and cooled gelatine or the agar-agar and then fold in the egg whites. Spoon the mixture over the base and smooth over. Chill in the deep-freeze for 15 minutes then transfer to the refrigerator until firmly set.

Loosen the cheesecake from the sides of the tin (pan) using a sharp knife and transfer it to a serving plate. Decorate the top with the finely grated lemon rind and serve or keep chilled until needed.

Panacotta with Pink Rhubarb

Only make this dish with forced pink rhubarb – otherwise, in order to get a nice pink colour, you will have to resort to tricks like adding redcurrant jelly to the poaching rhubarb or stirring in pink food colouring when the rhubarb is cooked.

Serves 6   GF   V

Panacotta

3 tablespoons cold filtered water

Scant tablespoon powdered gelatine (vegetarians use agar-agar)

125ml/½ cup creamy organic milk

450ml/1¾ cups organic double (heavy) cream

Pared rind of 1 small unwaxed orange

40g/⅓ cup unrefined icing (confectioners') sugar

2–3 tablespoons orange liqueur (coeliacs please check that the liqueur you use is suitable)

Rhubarb

680g/1½lbs forced pink rhubarb, trimmed and cut into bite-size chunks

Juice from the small orange used above

100g/½ cup unrefined golden caster (superfine) sugar

Optional

6 tiny sprigs of fresh mint

6 large individual tin pudding basins

Put the water in a glass bowl, sprinkle over the gelatine and leave to thicken for a few minutes.

Put the milk, 300ml/1¼ cups of the cream and the pared rind of the orange into a non-stick pan and bring to boiling point over medium heat. Remove from the heat immediately, stir the gelatine in and keep stirring until it dissolves. Cool and strain.

In a bowl, whisk the remaining cream, icing (confectioners') sugar and liqueur until lightly thickened. Fold in the cooled cream and pour the mixture into the moulds.

Refrigerate for 4 hours or until set. Meanwhile, put the rhubarb, orange juice and sugar in a pan and cook over low heat until the rhubarb is tender.

To serve the panacotta, dip the moulds into boiling water for a few seconds, ease a little bit of the dessert away from the tin using a little knife (to let the air in) and turn onto plates. Surround the panacotta with a little pool of the poached rhubarb and decorate with a tiny sprig of fresh mint.

Gâteau Paris-Brest

This is a classic French dessert, which you can buy in patisseries all over France.

Choux pastry is easy to make as long as you leave the mixture to cool before adding the eggs, otherwise the eggs start cooking too early and the pastry won't rise as much.

OPTIONAL

Serves 6

GF   V   DF

Choux pastry

55g/2oz organic butter or dairy-free margarine

125ml/½ cup cold filtered water

70g/½ cup organic rice flour, sifted onto a piece of baking parchment (wax paper)

2 organic free-range eggs, beaten

Filling

55g/⅓ cup unrefined golden caster (superfine) sugar

55g/scant ½ cup whole almonds

285ml/1⅓ cups organic double (heavy) cream, whipped

Icing (confectioners') sugar to dust

Optional

For dairy-free filling mix the praline with softened dairy-free vanilla ice cream and serve immediately

The Big Book of Wheat-Free Cooking

Preheat the oven to 220°C/420°F/Gas mark 7.

Make the choux pastry. Put the butter or margarine in a pan with the water and bring to the boil over medium heat. Once the fat has melted, remove the pan from the heat and immediately pour in the flour, beating until the mixture comes away from the sides of the pan. Leave to cool for about 10 minutes.

Gradually beat the eggs into the mixture until it is smooth and shiny; do not add all the egg if the mixture starts to lose its shape – it should be firm enough to hold its shape when spooned onto the baking tray.

Spoon the choux mixture into a ring about 18cm/7in wide on a dampened, non-stick baking sheet. Bake in the oven for 35 minutes. Transfer the ring to a wire rack and make small incisions into the side of the choux pastry to let out the steam.

Meanwhile, make the praline filling by slowly melting the sugar with the almonds in a pan, over low heat, stirring occasionally until it becomes dark caramel. Tip the hot mixture onto a lightly oiled baking tray and leave to cool. Once the praline has set, place in a plastic bag and bash it into tiny pieces using a rolling pin. Fold the cold praline into the whipped cream.

Carefully slice the choux ring in half horizontally, place on a serving dish and spoon in the filling. Cover with the top of the ring and dust with icing (confectioners') sugar.

You can serve the Gâteau Paris-Brest with warm chocolate sauce or a raspberry coulis. As an even more outrageous pudding, you can add sliced strawberries or fresh raspberries to the whipped cream – bliss!

Dark Chocolate Tart

This tart is perfection for a chocoholic, for any party or an Easter feast. A hint of cinnamon enhances the deep, dark flavour.

Serves 8

GF   **DF**

Pastry

200g/1¾ cups wheat-free flour mix*
125g/4½oz organic butter or dairy-free margarine, cut into small pieces
1 large organic free-range egg
Pinch of sea salt
A little cold water

Filling

3 large organic free-range eggs
4 large organic free-range egg yolks
60g/scant ⅓ cup unrefined golden caster (superfine) sugar
200g/7oz high quality bitter dark (bitter sweet) chocolate*, broken into pieces (this kind of chocolate should not have gluten or dairy in it but please check label)
150g/5oz organic butter or dairy-free margarine

25.5cm/10in non-stick loose-bottomed tart tin (pan)

* coeliacs please use gluten-free ingredients

Preheat the oven to 180°C/350°F/Gas mark 4.

Make the pastry by briefly blending the ingredients, except the water, in a food processor until it resembles breadcrumbs. Add a little water and whizz briefly until the pastry comes together into a ball of dough. Remove the pastry, wrap it in clingfilm (plastic wrap) and freeze for 10 minutes.

Roll out the pastry as thinly as possible on a floured board. Lift it over the tin (pan) and gently line with it. Put a circle of non-stick baking parchment (wax paper) on to the pastry base, fill with ceramic baking beans and bake blind for about 10 minutes. Remove the paper and ceramic baking beans and bake for a further 10 minutes.

Put the eggs, yolks and sugar into a big bowl and beat with an electric mixer on the highest speed for about 3 minutes until the mixture is pale, thick and creamy.

Melt the chocolate and margarine together either in a bowl in the microwave or in a bowl set over a pan of simmering water. Stir the chocolate until smooth and then scrape every bit of it into the egg mixture. Beat with a wooden spoon until blended and then pour into the pastry case. Bake in the oven for about 15 minutes, or until the filling is nearly set, and then leave it to cool. Transfer to a serving plate and serve at room temperature.

Rhubarb and Oatmeal Possets

Possets started as warm ale curdled with boiling milk but by the mid-18th century they were made with cream and sack (sweet sherry). Elizabeth Moxon's version from the book English Housewifery *(1749) used cream, white wine, lemon zest and whisked egg whites. Here is a more contemporary version for the 21st century.*

Serves 4

V   Q&E

455g/1lb trimmed cultivated pink rhubarb stems, chopped into bite-size pieces
4 tablespoons unrefined golden granulated sugar
60ml/¼ cup good quality white wine
3 tablespoons fine organic porridge oats (oatmeal)
A sprinkling of ground cinnamon
310ml/1¼ cups organic double (heavy) cream
Finely grated rind of ½ small, unwaxed lemon
1 large organic free-range egg white, whisked until stiff

Place the rhubarb, half the sugar and all the wine in a pan and simmer over low heat until soft. Meanwhile, mix the oats (oatmeal), the remaining sugar and the cinnamon together and sprinkle over a non-stick baking tray. Grill (broil) until golden, then toss and turn the crumbs and cook until dark golden. Cool until needed and then break it up into flaky caramelized pieces.

Allow the rhubarb to cool, blend it to a purée and then transfer to a large bowl. Whip the cream in a bowl and fold it into the purée with the finely grated lemon rind and lastly the whisked egg white. Divide the mixture between 4 wine glasses and level off. Sprinkle the tops with the oats (oatmeal) and chill until needed. The possets must be served on the day of making.

Passion Cakes with Passion Sauce

A romantic at heart, I need no excuse to create a special feast for St Valentine's Day or even just a quiet, cosy, candlelit dinner together to make the person you care for feel extra special. Heart-shaped tins (pans) are available from all good cook shops, some of which do mail order as well.

Serves 2–4

GF   DF   V

60g/⅔ cup ground almonds

30g/¼ cup wheat-free flour* mix, sifted

2 large organic free-range eggs, separated

75g/⅔ cup unrefined golden caster (superfine) sugar

1 teaspoon bitter almond extract

Flesh and juice of 6 ripe passion fruit (the more wrinkled they are, the riper)

Sprinkling of sifted unrefined icing (confectioners') sugar

Juice of ½ a small lemon

4 tablespoons Archers Peach Schnapps

Little exotic flowers or tiny sprigs of mint, if available, for decoration

---

4 heart-shaped baking moulds about 9.5cm/3¾ in in length lined with non-stick baking parchment (wax paper)

---

* coeliacs please use gluten-free ingredients

Preheat the oven to 180°C/350°F/Gas mark 4.

Mix the ground almonds with the flour in a bowl. In the food processor, beat the egg yolks and sugar with the almond extract until pale and thick. Scrape the egg mixture out of the food processor and stir it into the flour. Quickly slice open 2 of the passion fruits, scoop the filling out and pour into the flour mixture.

Beat the egg whites into soft peaks and fold into the passion fruit mixture. Divide the mixture between the prepared heart moulds and bake for about 15 minutes until golden and springy to touch. Leave them to cool slightly and then turn them onto wire racks.

Just before serving, place one heart on each plate and dust with icing (confectioners') sugar. Halve each of the remaining passion fruit; scoop the flesh out and into a small bowl. Stir in some of the lemon juice and all the peach schnapps. Taste to see if any more lemon juice is needed. Spoon the passion sauce over the pointed tip of each heart and into a little pool. Decorate with a flower or a few tiny sprigs of fresh mint.

Raspberry and Pecan Roulade

Nuts, raspberries and cream are such a divine combination. In this recipe the roulade is made rather more slimming by using fromage frais. Consequently, we can allow ourselves the occasional indulgence when entertaining friends or family.

GF   V

Serves 8

4 large organic eggs, separated

Finely grated rind of 1 unwaxed orange

110g/½ cup unrefined golden caster (superfine) sugar, plus extra for sprinkling

Juice of ½ an orange

110g/4oz pack walnuts or pecan nuts, chopped very finely

500g/2 cups strawberry flavour virtually fat-free fromage frais

225g/½lb fresh, ripe raspberries

Swiss roll/roulade tin (pan), about 28 x 38cm/11 x 15in, lined with non-stick baking parchment (wax paper)

The Big Book of Wheat-Free Cooking

Preheat the oven to 170°C/325°F/Gas mark 3.

Put the egg yolks and the grated orange rind into a large bowl and whisk briefly with an electric whisk. Add 75g/⅓ cup of sugar and beat at high speed until thick and light, about 3 minutes. Add the orange juice, whisk on the highest speed for another 2 minutes and then fold in the nuts.

In a separate bowl, whisk the egg whites until stiff, adding the remaining sugar until you have firm peaks. Fold the egg whites lightly into the nut mixture. Spread this quickly and evenly over the prepared tray.

Place the roulade in the middle of the oven for 15 minutes, until golden brown all over and just springy when lightly pressed with your fingertips. While the roulade is cooking, spread another similar sized piece of non-stick baking parchment (wax paper) on to the work surface and sprinkle it lightly with a little caster (superfine) sugar.

Remove the roulade from the oven and turn it out on to the sugared paper. Carefully peel the paper away from the roulade and discard it. Cover the roulade with a clean tea towel and leave to cool.

Spread the fromage frais over the cold sponge, sprinkle the raspberries over the roulade and roll up. The easiest way is to take both corners of the short edge of parchment and gently roll the first third over the second, peel away the paper and flip the roulade on to the serving dish. Cover and keep chilled until needed. I make this a day in advance and it is just as good.

Peach Angel Ring with Strawberry Coulis

This is such a delicious summer combination, with distant memories of the peach melba that we used to love as children. You can also use nectarines, but apricots are a little too dry for them to be a success.

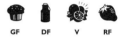

Serves 8–12

GF **DF** **V** **RF**

Cake

125g/1 cup wheat-free flour mix*

185g/1 scant cup unrefined golden caster (superfine) sugar

Pinch of sea salt

7 large organic free-range egg whites

2 teaspoons cream of tartar

1 tablespoon Archers Peach Schnapps

Peach filling and strawberry coulis

4–6 ripe peaches, peeled, halved, stoned (pitted) and thickly sliced

850g/3½ pints ripe strawberries, hulled and wiped clean (or frozen and defrosted)

2 tablespoons rosewater

A large, deep, non-stick ring baking tin (pan) or a large, deep, non-stick Kugelhupf mould

* coeliacs please use gluten-free ingredients

Preheat the oven to 180°C/350°F/Gas mark 4.

First make the cake. Sift together the flour, 7 tablespoons of the sugar and the salt in a bowl and set aside. In another larger bowl, whisk the egg whites at medium speed for 2 minutes, or until they are thick and foamy. Add the cream of tartar and increase the speed to high. Slowly sprinkle the remaining sugar into the egg whites and beat them until they form soft peaks. Add the peach schnapps and fold in the sugar and sifted flour mixture. Pour the cake mixture into the tin (pan) and bake in the oven for about 40 minutes, or until an inserted skewer comes out clean. The cake should be golden and firm to touch. Leave the cake to cool in the tin (pan) for 20 minutes, after which time the cake should come away from the sides.

Ease the cake out and turn it on to a large serving plate. Fill the centre of the cake with the prepared peaches so that it looks pretty.

To make the coulis, put the strawberries and rosewater into the food processor and pulse to a purée. Press the coulis through a fine sieve and discard the pips. The sauce should be thick, but just runny enough to spoon over the cake so that it trickles down the sides. Spoon some of the coulis on to the fruit and cake. Serve the rest of the sauce separately.

Blackberry and Apple Tartlets

A walk in the country can be full of hidden treasures such as wild blackberries growing rampantly in the hedgerows and old orchard apples, which have tumbled to the ground, ripe and ready to eat. Make sure both fruits are ripe and juicy and then the recipe will be even more delicious.

Serves 8–16

GF   DF   V

Pastry

200g/1¾ cups wheat-free flour mix*
125g/4½oz organic butter or dairy-free margarine, cut into 5 pieces
1 large organic free-range egg
Pinch of sea salt
A little cold water

Filling

1kg/2½lbs sweet eating apples
255g/1½ cups ripe blackberries without any stalks
Finely grated rind and juice of 1 unwaxed lemon
Pinch of ground cloves
Sprinkling of unrefined golden caster (superfine) sugar

12-cup tartlet tray lined with non-stick paper circles (this is not necessary if it is a non-stick tray)

* coeliacs please use gluten-free ingredients

Preheat the oven to 180°C/350°F/Gas mark 4.

Make the pastry by briefly blending the ingredients, except the water, in a food processor until it resembles breadcrumbs. Add a little water and whizz briefly until the pastry comes together into a ball of dough. Remove the pastry, wrap it in clingfilm (plastic wrap) and freeze for 10 minutes.

Using a lemon zester, peel thin strips of rind off the lemon and keep for decorating the tarts later on.

Peel, quarter and remove the cores from the apples and thinly slice them into a pan with the lemon juice and the ground cloves. Simmer over a low heat until soft, stirring occasionally – this takes about 20 minutes. Gently stir in the blackberries and remove from the heat.

Roll out the pastry thinly enough on a floured board so that you can cut out about 16 circles with a suitable-sized fluted cutter. Line 12 of the cups with the pastry and prick the bases with a fork. Fill them with the blackberry and apple mixture, sprinkle with a little caster (superfine) sugar and bake in the oven for about 25 minutes until the pastry is golden. Leave them to cool and then carefully lift them out of the tray and on to a serving dish or wire rack. Make the remaining tarts in the same way.

Serve the tarts at room temperature, decorated with a pinch of the lemon peel. They are delicious on their own, but some guests may like a bowl of virtually fat-free fromage frais or soya vanilla ice cream to delve into.

Warm Desserts ...

Baked Alaska

To make this dessert extra special, you can macerate the fruit overnight in a complementary liqueur. If you want to make your own sponge and freeze it for a later date then this pudding can be assembled very quickly. You can also use a bag of frozen mixed berries if fresh fruit is out of season.

OPTIONAL

Serves 6–8

V   GF   DF

280g/10oz Village Bakery organic wheat-free lemon cake or you can use a wheat-free vanilla or Madeira cake (for gluten- and dairy-free choose another brand or make your own)

1 litre/4 cups of a complementary ice cream such as lemon, vanilla, pecan toffee crunch or pralines and cream – make sure it is wheat or gluten free (Tofutti dairy-free ice cream can be used instead – see page 305 for stockist)

4 large organic free-range egg whites

225g/8oz unrefined golden caster (superfine) sugar

500g/1lb 2oz mixed summer berries, such as raspberries, strawberries and blueberries, or defrost and drain frozen fruit

Preheat the oven to 220°C/425°F/Gas mark 7.

Cut the cake in half widthways then cut each half lengthways into 3 slices. Lay the cake slices on a flat and shallow ovenproof dish to form one large rectangle.

If the ice cream is not quite soft enough let it sit for 10 minutes and then ease it out. Mould the ice cream over the sponge to form a rectangle, leaving a 1cm/½ in border around the edge of the sponge.

Place in the freezer and freeze for about 30–50 minutes.

In a large bowl, whisk the egg whites into soft peaks and then whisk in the sugar, a couple of tablespoons at a time, until the mixture is stiff and glossy. Take the ice cream cake out of the freezer and quickly cover it with the fruit and then the meringue. Swirl the meringue into peaks, making sure you enclose the cake completely in meringue. Bake for about 5–10 minutes until the meringue is golden brown with dark ridges – keep peeping into the oven to check the meringue doesn't burn. Serve the Baked Alaska immediately.

The Big Book of Wheat-Free Cooking

Foolproof Boozy Custard

This custard is perfect with any pudding but it is particularly good with Christmas pudding if you don't like brandy butter. Custard doesn't freeze but it is quick to make and you can keep it in the refrigerator for a couple of days – but be careful not to boil it when you reheat it.

Serves 8

GF   DF   V

625ml/2½ cups organic milk or organic dairy-free Provamel vanilla soya milk

1 vanilla pod, cut and opened out lengthways or 2 teaspoons vanilla extract

4 large organic free-range egg yolks

90g/scant ½ cup unrefined golden caster (superfine) sugar

2 tablespoons pure cornflour (cornstarch)

2 tablespoons good brandy, dark rum or Marsala

125ml/½ cup organic double (heavy) cream or Provamel Soya Dream

---

Pour the milk into a non-stick pan, add the vanilla pod and simmer gently over low heat until the milk reaches boiling point. Meanwhile, put the egg yolks, sugar and cornflour (cornstarch) into a food processor and blend until pale and smooth. Remove the pan from the heat and leave to cool for 5 minutes before removing the vanilla pod.

With the food processor running, pour in the milk and mix thoroughly. Add the vanilla extract if you haven't used a pod and give the custard a brief whiz.

Transfer the custard back to the pan and cook over low heat, stirring all the time, until thick and smooth. Remove the custard from the heat as it reaches boiling point. Stir in the cream and then brandy, one spoon at a time, and transfer the custard to a warm jug or bowl to serve.

If you wish to set the custard aside for later use, pour and scrape it into a bowl, cover the surface of the custard with greased non-stick baking parchment (wax paper) and cool, cover and chill it until needed.

Ten-minute Chocolate Puddings

These puddings only take 10 minutes to cook, hence the name. They're simple to make and will impress everybody. Serve the puddings with crème fraîche or a dairy-free alternative or on their own.

GF   DF   V   Q&E

Serves 6

185g/6½oz dark dairy-free chocolate (73% pure cocoa is excellent), broken into pieces
185g/6½oz organic butter or dairy-free margarine, plus extra for greasing
3 organic free-range eggs plus 3 extra egg yolks
6 tablespoons unrefined golden caster (superfine) sugar
3 teaspoons wheat-free flour mix*
Sieved cocoa powder for dusting*

Optional
Crème fraîche or Provamel dairy-free Soya Dream to serve

6 large individual tin pudding moulds, fluted moulds or large ramekins lined with a circle of baking parchment (wax paper)

---

* *coeliacs please use gluten-free ingredients*

Preheat the oven to 220°C/425°F/Gas mark 7.

Melt the chocolate and butter or margarine in a heatproof bowl over a pan of simmering water, stirring occasionally until smooth and glossy.

In a separate bowl, whisk the eggs, yolks and sugar until thickened. Whisk in the melted chocolate mixture and sieve and fold in the flour. Divide the mixture between the prepared moulds.

Bake the puddings for 9–10 minutes until the outside is set but the inside is still soft.

Carefully turn each pudding out onto a warm plate and serve with a dusting of cocoa powder and, if you want, a dollop of crème fraîche or Soya Dream.

Cherry Rum Puddings

Rum-soaked dried cherries or cranberries make this a cheerful and filling winter pudding. Serve the puddings with the Foolproof Boozy Custard on page 237.

GF DF V

Makes 6

5 tablespoons dark rum

75g/⅔ cup dried cherries or cranberries

170g/6oz organic butter or dairy-free margarine

170g/¾ cup unrefined golden caster (superfine) sugar

3 organic free-range eggs, beaten

140g/1 heaped cup wheat-free flour mix*

2 teaspoons wheat-free baking powder*

55g/⅔ cup ground almonds

55g/2oz fresh white wheat-free breadcrumbs* (see page 305 for stockist)

6 large individual tin pudding basins, generously greased and lined with a circle of baking parchment (wax paper) or Bake-O-Glide

* coeliacs please use gluten-free ingredients

Preheat the oven to 180°C/350°F/Gas mark 4.

Heat the rum in a small pan and add the cherries or cranberries. Stir, remove from the heat and leave to soak for 1 hour.

Beat the butter or margarine and sugar together in a food processor until light and fluffy. Briefly beat in the eggs and the flour and then transfer to a bowl. Fold in the baking powder, almonds, breadcrumbs and lastly the cherries and rum.

Spoon the mixture into the prepared moulds and level off the surface. Loosely place a circle of baking parchment (wax paper) on the top and then seal with a circle of kitchen foil.

Place the moulds in a large roasting pan half full of hot water and bake for about 40 minutes until a skewer, inserted into the pudding, comes out clean.

Turn the pudding out onto warm plates and serve with warm wheat- and gluten-free custard.

Spiced Bread Pudding

This pudding is not a traditional bread and butter pudding but it is another equally old and traditional recipe. The pudding uses up stale bread instead of fresh bread and is spicy and rich.

Serves 6

DF   V

115g/¾ cup sultanas (golden raisins)

30g/¼ cup currants

30g/¼ cup raisins or mixed peel

3 tablespoons dark rum

250g/9oz trimmed weight of fresh The Village Bakery Raisin Borodinsky rye bread or other wheat-free fruity
   rye bread if this isn't available (see page 304 for stockist)

375ml/1½ cups organic milk or Provamel organic vanilla soya milk

55g/2oz organic butter or dairy-free margarine, plus a little extra for greasing

85g/½ cup unrefined dark soft brown sugar

2 teaspoons mixed spice (pie spice)*

1 large organic free-range egg, beaten

Finely grated rind of 1 unwaxed orange or lemon

Freshly grated nutmeg

1 heaped tablespoon unrefined demerara sugar

23cm/9in square, ovenproof serving dish with deep sides, greased

---

* coeliacs please use gluten-free ingredients

Preheat the oven to 180°C/350°F/Gas mark 4.

Put all the dried fruits in a bowl with the rum and leave to marinate for as long as you like during the day.

When you are ready to make the pudding, cut the bread into 6 slices and then into quarters. Put the bread into a bowl, pour over the milk and leave for 30 minutes.

Meanwhile, over low heat, melt the butter or margarine in a pan with the sugar and mixed spice (pie spice). Remove from the heat, transfer to a large bowl, stir in the beaten egg and marinated fruits and rum. Stir in the finely grated orange or lemon rind and gently combine with the bread and milk.

Pour the mixture into the prepared dish, level off the bread and sprinkle with grated nutmeg and demerara sugar. Bake for about 50 minutes until puffy and golden around the edges.

Serve warm with crème fraîche, dairy-free vanilla ice cream or, for the ultimate wickedness, the Marmalade Ice Cream recipe on page 214.

Individual Queen of Puddings

The joy of this classic English pudding is that it uses everyday ingredients – butter, milk, bread, eggs and any flavour jam (jelly) you like. Usually queen of puddings is served in one dish – which is great for Sunday lunch – but as individual puddings they are more fun and perfect for winter dinner parties.

Serves 6

GF   DF   V   Q&E

580ml/2⅓ cups organic milk or Provamel organic vanilla soya milk

20g/¾oz organic butter or dairy-free margarine and a little extra for greasing

130g/1½ cups fresh gluten-free white breadcrumbs* (see page 305 for stockist)

110g/½ cup unrefined golden caster (superfine) sugar, plus 1 extra teaspoon for the tops

Finely grated rind of 1 unwaxed lemon

3 large organic free-range eggs, separated

6 tablespoons Morello cherry conserve, or any other favourite jam (jelly), warmed in a pan

6 large ramekins, generously greased

* coeliacs please use gluten-free ingredients

Preheat oven to 180°C/350°F/Gas mark 4.

Bring the milk to the boil in a non-stick pan, remove from the heat and stir in the butter or margarine, breadcrumbs, 55g/¼ cup of the sugar and the grated lemon rind. Leave to one side for 20 minutes to allow the crumbs to swell.

Separate the eggs into two bowls. Beat the egg yolks and stir into the crumb mixture. Divide the mixture between the ramekins and level off. Place on a baking tray and bake for about 25 minutes until set. Remove the ramekins from the oven and put one spoonful of the jam (jelly) in each one. If you put too much jam (jelly) in, it will overflow.

Whisk the egg whites until stiff and fold in the remaining sugar. Divide the meringue between the ramekins, piling it up into swirly peaks. Sprinkle the teaspoon of sugar over the tops.

Return the puddings to the oven and bake for about 10 minutes until golden brown. The puddings will keep warm whilst you finish your main course.

Baked Apples with Spiced Cranberry Stuffing

If you have a sweet tooth you can add a little more honey or maple syrup to the recipe.

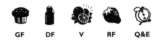

Serves 2 (double the ingredients for the menu on page 297)

GF   DF   V   RF   Q&E

2 large cooking apples, central core removed (pulled out without splitting the apple)
40g/⅔ cup dried cranberries or 85g/3oz fresh, frozen (partly defrosted) cranberries
1 heaped teaspoon freshly grated root ginger
Finely grated rind of ½ an unwaxed orange
½ teaspoon mixed spice* (pie spice)
2 tablespoons runny honey or organic maple syrup

*coeliacs please use gluten-free ingredients

Preheat the oven to 180°C/350°F/Gas mark 4.

Place the cored apples, so that they do not touch, in a small ovenproof baking and serving dish. In a small bowl, mix the cranberries with the ginger, orange rind, mixed spice (pie spice) and honey or syrup. Pack it right down into the cavity of each apple so that it touches the base of the dish. It is easier to start spooning the mixture using a teaspoon and finish pushing it down using clean fingertips. Let the remaining fresh cranberries tumble over the tops of the apples.

Spoon 1 tablespoon of cold water into the dish, but not over the apples, and bake for about 25–30 minutes or until the apples are puffy and cooked through, but not to the point of collapse or bursting. Leave them to cool slightly in the dish, then transfer to warm plates with any juices, and serve.

Prune, Almond and Cognac Tart

This is my winter favourite. The luscious combination of prunes, almonds and cognac matches well with warming winter game dishes or Sunday roasts. Because the mixture works so well, I have never tried an alternative to the prunes but if you are not a great fan, then I suggest you try ready-to-eat figs and prepare the tart in the same way.

Serves 6–8

GF   V

Pastry

200g/1¾ cups wheat-free flour mix*
125g/4½oz organic butter, cut into 6 pieces
Pinch of sea salt
1 organic free-range egg
A little cold water

Filling

4 heaped tablespoons half-fat crème fraîche
2 large organic free-range eggs
120g/¾ cup unrefined golden caster (superfine) sugar
125g/generous 1¼ cups ground almonds
4 tablespoons cognac
1 teaspoon pure bitter almond oil or extract
60g/4 tablespoons organic butter
30 ready-to-eat stoned (pitted) prunes – if they are unavailable, use normal prunes, put them in a bowl of boiling weak tea to cover and let them soak overnight

25.5cm/10in round, loose-bottomed, non-stick, fluted tart tin (pan)

coeliacs please use gluten-free ingredients

Preheat the oven to 180°C/350°F/Gas mark 4.

Make the pastry in the food processor. Put in the pastry ingredients, except the water, and whizz for a few seconds until the mixture resembles breadcrumbs. Cautiously add the water and process briefly until it comes together into a ball of dough. Remove the dough, wrap it in clingfilm (plastic wrap) and freeze for 10 minutes. Roll out the dough thinly on a floured board and line the baking tin (pan).

Beat together the crème fraîche, eggs, sugar, almonds, half the cognac and the almond oil in the food processor for a few seconds. Melt the butter in a small bowl in the microwave or in a small saucepan over a medium heat. Briefly beat the butter into the mixture.

Drain and discard the liquid from the prunes, arrange them over the pastry base and then pour over the almond mixture. Bake the tart for 30 minutes, remove from the oven and sprinkle with the remaining cognac. Allow the tin (pan) to cool so that you can carefully lift the tart out on to a serving dish.

Pumpkin Pie

You can use fresh or canned pumpkin for this recipe, according to the amount of time – and space – you have available. If you have children, it is great entertainment for them to scoop out the flesh of the pumpkin and make funny masks for Halloween.

GF   DF   V

Serves 6–8

Pastry

200g/1¾ cups wheat-free flour mix*
125g/4½oz organic butter or dairy-free margarine, cut into 8 pieces
Pinch of sea salt
1 organic free-range egg
A little cold water

Filling

200ml/¾ cup bottled, freshly pressed apple juice
1 tablespoon pure cornflour (cornstarch)
425g/scant 2 cups canned or freshly cooked pumpkin flesh, mashed until smooth
2 large organic free-range eggs, beaten
3 heaped teaspoons peeled and coarsely grated root ginger
4 tablespoons organic maple syrup
1 teaspoon mixed spice* (pie spice)
1 teaspoon ground cinnamon
A pinch of ground cloves
A little freshly grated nutmeg

25.5cm/10in fluted, loose-bottomed tart tin (pan)

coeliacs please use gluten-free ingredients

Preheat the oven to 180°C/350°F/Gas mark 4.

First make the pastry. Put all the ingredients, except the water, into a food processor and whizz for a few seconds until the mixture resembles breadcrumbs. Cautiously add the water and process briefly until it comes together into a ball of dough. Remove the dough, wrap it in clingfilm (plastic wrap) and freeze for 10 minutes.

Roll out the dough on a floured board into a medium–thick pastry and then lift it over the baking dish and line it. Press it gently down to fit the dish, cutting away any remnants hanging over the sides. Prick the base with a fork and leave to one side while you make the filling.

Mix the apple juice and the cornflour (cornstarch) together in a small bowl. Put the pumpkin flesh into a larger bowl and then stir in the apple juice mixture. Mix in the eggs, ginger, maple syrup and all the spices. When the mixture is smooth, spoon it into the prepared pastry case. Level it off and bake the pie for about 35 minutes until the filling is set and firm and the pastry is golden. Serve the pumpkin pie warm.

Cakes and Cookies ...

Gooseberry Sauce Cake

You can use whatever stewed fruit is in season for this delicious cake, and add or deduct sugar according to how sweet your chosen fruit is. In winter I use canned gooseberries, drained.

Serves 8

GF **DF** **V**

285g/2½ cups wheat-free flour mix*
3 teaspoons wheat-free baking powder*
½ teaspoon fine salt
170g/¾ cup unrefined golden caster (superfine) sugar
115g/4oz organic butter or dairy-free margarine, melted
2 large organic free-range eggs
400ml/2 cups unsweetened stewed gooseberries
1 teaspoon pure vanilla extract
2 tablespoons unrefined demerara sugar

23cm/9in cake tin (pan), greased and lined with non-stick baking parchment (wax paper) or Bake-O-Glide

* coeliacs please use gluten-free ingredients

Preheat the oven to 180°C/350°F/Gas mark 4.

In a bowl, mix the flour with the baking powder, salt and caster (superfine) sugar. Make a well in the centre and add the melted butter or dairy-free margarine, eggs, gooseberries and vanilla.

Combine the mixture thoroughly and spoon it into the prepared tin (pan). Smooth the surface and sprinkle with the demerara sugar.

Bake for about 45 minutes until firm to touch with the tip of your fingers. You can also test if the cake is done by inserting a skewer; if it comes out clean, the cake is cooked.

Let the cake cool in the tin (pan) before turning out onto a serving plate. The cake is delicious served with half fat crème fraîche or dairy-free Tofutti Sour Supreme.

Christmas Mincemeat Torte

This torte is brilliant because you can change the filling to suit the season – you can use mincemeat at Christmas, blackcurrants in summer and cherries in the spring.

Serves 6–8

GF   DF   V

170g/6oz organic butter or dairy-free margarine, softened

170g/¾ cup unrefined golden caster (superfine) sugar

170g/1⅓ cups Orgran self-raising wheat-free flour*

A pinch of fine salt

170g/1⅔ cups ground almonds

A pinch of ground cinnamon if desired

2 organic free-range eggs and 1 egg yolk

415g/15oz jar vegetarian luxury mincemeat

A little sieved unrefined icing (confectioners') sugar

23cm/9in round, loose-bottomed, spring-clip cake tin (pan), lined with a circle of non-stick baking parchment (wax paper) or Bake-O-Glide

* coeliacs please use gluten-free ingredients

Preheat the oven to 180°C/350°F/Gas mark 4.

Put the butter, sugar, flour, salt, almonds, cinnamon, eggs and egg yolk in a food processor and blend until just combined.

Gently spread half the mixture in the base of the tin (pan), using clean fingertips or two forks. Lightly spread the mincemeat over the mixture but not too near the edge. Now gently spread the remaining mixture over the mincemeat, using clean fingertips or the forks. Don't worry about a few gaps.

Bake for about 50 minutes until well-risen and golden brown. Cool in the tin (pan) for about half an hour and then carefully remove the tin (pan) and slide the torte onto a plate. Dust with a little icing (confectioners') sugar and serve.

Creole Christmas Cake

This cake makes a nice change from the more usual British Christmas cake and has a less formal look to it. Provided you don't ice the cake, it will keep for one month in an airtight container or up to 3 months in the freezer – simply open-freeze it and then wrap it in clingfilm (plastic wrap). Thaw the cake in a cool place overnight. The iced cake will keep for up to a week.

Serves about 16–20   GF   DF   V

2 days in advance soak the following fruit in 250ml/1 cup of dark rum:

175g/1 heaped cup pitted prunes, coarsely chopped

175g/1 heaped cup raisins

175g/1 heaped cup currants

125g/scant cup natural glacé cherries, halved

100g/scant cup chopped candied peel

170g/6oz organic butter, softened, or dairy-free margarine

170g/1¼ cups dark molasses (dark soft brown) sugar

4 organic free-range eggs, beaten

100g/¾ cup organic buckwheat flour

100g/¾ cup organic rice flour

3 heaped tablespoons molasses

2 teaspoons ground allspice

85g/scant ½ cup stem ginger pieces, chopped

2 heaped teaspoons wheat-free baking powder*

Icing

455g/1lb unrefined icing (confectioners') sugar

3 tablespoons stem ginger syrup

55g/2oz organic butter or dairy-free margarine

3 tablespoons dark rum

Optional

30g/¼ cup dried cranberries to decorate or other festive allergy-free decorations

20.5cm/8in round, deep cake tin (pan), greased and sides and base lined with non-stick baking parchment (wax paper) or Bake-O-Glide

---

* coeliacs please use gluten-free ingredients

Preheat the oven to 150°C/300°F/Gas mark 2.

Keep the fruit covered and cool while it soaks.

Beat together the butter or margarine with the sugar until smooth and creamy. Beat in some of the egg and then some of the flour, alternating until both ingredients are used up. Mix in the soaked fruit and rum and then stir in the molasses. Stir in the allspice, ginger and baking powder. Spoon the mixture into the prepared tin (pan) and bake for 3 hours. You can test if it is cooked by inserting a skewer into the centre of the cake – if it comes out clean the cake is cooked through.

Cool the cake for 1 hour in the tin (pan) and then turn it out onto a wire rack to cool completely.

Beat the icing ingredients together in a bowl with an electric whisk until the mixture is smooth and creamy. Put the cake onto a serving plate and swirl the icing all over the cake using a spatula.

If you wish, you can decorate the cake with a sprinkling of dried cranberries before serving.

Apple and Lemon Streusel Cake

This pudding can be made a day in advance and reheated when needed. You can replace the Kirsch with any liqueur that you fancy – provided it is gluten- and dairy-free if necessary – and you could replace the apples with pears for a change.

GF   **DF**   **V**

Serves 8

650g/1lb 7oz peeled and cored dessert apples, diced
Finely grated rind of 1 unwaxed lemon
250g/2 cups wheat-free flour mix*
3 teaspoons wheat-free baking powder*
Pinch of fine salt
115g/4oz organic butter or dairy-free margarine
200g/1 cup unrefined golden caster (superfine) sugar
½ teaspoon pure vanilla extract
2 large organic free-range eggs
2 tablespoons organic milk or organic unsweetened dairy-free soya milk

Streusel topping

30g/1oz organic butter or dairy-free margarine, chilled
55g/½ cup wheat-free flour mix*
55g/⅓ cup unrefined demerara sugar
2 tablespoons roasted hazelnuts, chopped
Finely grated rind of 2 unwaxed lemons
A good pinch of ground cinnamon

Optional

Crème fraîche or dairy-free vanilla ice cream to serve

23cm/9in spring-form, loose-bottomed cake tin (pan), greased all over and lined with a circle of baking
   parchment (wax paper) or Bake-O-Glide

* coeliacs please use gluten-free ingredients

Preheat the oven to 180°C/350°F/Gas mark 4.

Mix the apples with the lemon juice and rind. Sift the flour into a bowl along with the baking powder and salt. In another bowl, beat the butter or margarine and sugar together with the vanilla extract. Now mix in the eggs and fold in the flour mixture, milk and apples. Set aside while you make the topping.

Rub the butter or margarine into the flour to make fine crumbs and then mix in the remaining topping ingredients.

Spoon the cake mixture into the tin (pan) and level off. Sprinkle on the topping. Bake for about 1 hour 10 minutes until golden and firm to the touch. Cool the cake for 20 minutes before turning it out onto a warm serving dish. Serve with crème fraîche or dairy-free vanilla ice cream.

Marbled Cherry and Almond Cake

You can freeze this cake but it also stores well wrapped in foil and kept in a cool place for up to a week. This cake is excellent for making the Cranberry Trifle on page 204.

GF **DF** **V**

Serves 12

155g/1⅓ cups Orgran gluten-free self-raising flour (see page 305 for stockist)
100g/3½oz packet ground almonds
170g/6oz organic butter or organic dairy-free margarine
155g/¾ cup unrefined golden caster (superfine) sugar
2 organic free-range eggs, beaten
Few drops of pure almond extract
4 tablespoons organic milk or unsweetened dairy-free organic soya milk
155g/½ cup black cherry jam (jelly)
30g/⅓ cup flaked almonds

900g/2lb loaf tin (pan), greased and lined with baking parchment (wax paper)

Preheat oven to 170°C/325°F/Gas mark 3.

Beat the flour, almonds, butter or margarine, sugar, eggs, almond extract and milk together in a food processor until light and fluffy. Spoon half this mixture into the prepared tin (pan) and spoon the jam (jelly) evenly over the top. Cover with the remaining cake mixture, then, using a skewer, swirl the jam (jelly) through the mixture. Smooth the top, scatter with the almonds and bake for about 1 hour until firm to touch.

Leave the cake in the tin (pan) until cool, turn out onto a wire rack and leave until cold. Serve sliced or freeze whole.

Porter Cake

Porter cake is usually made with the black stout of Ireland, which makes it very rich and moist. You can, however, use any beer, stout or lager, depending on your loyalties!

Serves 8

DF   V

455g/1lb wheat-free flour mix*
A pinch of fine salt
2 teaspoons wheat-free baking powder*
225g/generous cup unrefined golden caster (superfine) sugar
1 teaspoon nutmeg, freshly grated
2 teaspoons mixed spice (pie spice)*
225g/8oz organic butter or dairy-free margarine
455g/1lb sultanas (golden raisins)
55g/2oz candied peel
55g/2oz glacé cherries
4400ml/1¾ cups stout, ale or lager
2 large organic free-range eggs, beaten

20.5cm/8in non-stick cake tin (pan) lined with baking parchment (wax paper) or Bake-O-Glide

* coeliacs please use gluten-free ingredients

Preheat the oven to 180°C/350°F/Gas mark 4.

Sieve the flour, salt and baking powder into a bowl and then add the sugar, nutmeg and spice. Rub the butter or margarine in with your fingertips, then gently stir in the fruit, stout and beaten eggs.

Turn the mixture into the prepared tin (pan) and bake for about 2 hours in the oven. Cool in the tin (pan), then remove it and wrap in baking parchment (wax paper) and clingfilm (plastic wrap). Keep for 3 days before eating.

Chocolate Almond Gâteau

This incredibly rich cake is perfect for special anniversaries or christenings or can be served as a decadent dessert for a dinner or lunch party. Use the best chocolate that you can find – Valrhona, El Rey, and Menier are all excellent but make sure that whichever variety you use, the cocoa content is at least 72%. You can make this gâteau about three to four days in advance.

GF   DF   V

Serves 8

170g/6oz El Rey dark chocolate (73.5% cocoa) or other dairy-free brands*

3 tablespoons Jamaica rum

85g/¾ cup whole almonds

170g/6oz organic butter or dairy-free margarine

170g/6oz unrefined golden caster (superfine) sugar plus 2 tablespoons for the egg whites

5 organic free-range eggs, separated

Chocolate icing

170g/6oz El Rey dark chocolate (dairy-free)

3 tablespoons Jamaica rum

170g/6oz organic butter or dairy-free margarine

55g/2oz unrefined golden granulated sugar

Optional decorations

Crystallized violets for special occasions or whole, skinned almonds for other occasions

2 x 20.5cm/8in cake tins (pans), base and sides lined with circles of baking parchment (wax paper) or Bake-O-Glide

---

The Big Book of Wheat-Free Cooking

Preheat the oven to 180°C/350°F/Gas mark 4.

Melt the chocolate with the rum in a bowl over a pan of simmering water. Grind the almonds in a blender but not to the extent that they become a powder. In a large bowl, beat the butter or margarine with the caster (superfine) sugar until light and fluffy and then beat in the egg yolks one by one. Stir the melted chocolate and rum into the butter mixture and then stir in the almonds.

Whisk the egg whites in another bowl until stiff. Add the 2 tablespoons of sugar and whisk until stiff peaks form. Lightly fold the egg whites into the chocolate mixture until well combined.

Divide the mixture between the two tins (pans), making a hollow in the centre of each cake. Bake the cakes in the oven for about 20 minutes – they should be slightly underdone in the middle. Leave the cakes to cool in the tins (pans).

Meanwhile, make the icing. Melt the chocolate with the rum in a bowl over a pan of simmering water. Whisk in the butter or margarine, a little at a time, and remove from the heat. Whisk in the sugar and stir the icing from time to time as it cools.

When the cakes are cold, place one top side down, on a serving plate and spread with icing; top with the remaining cake, top side up, and cover the whole cake with icing. Leave enough icing to pipe around the top of the cake. Decorate with whole almonds or, for special occasions, with crystallized violets or a combination of both.

Almond and Chocolate Chip Cake

I love these all-in-one-mix cakes, as they make life so much simpler if you are expecting friends or have hungry children coming to tea. This cake freezes beautifully wrapped in slices, which is ideal for a school or work lunchbox.

GF   DF   V

Serves 10

200g/2 cups wheat-free flour mix*

2 teaspoons wheat-free baking powder*

170g/6oz organic soft margarine or dairy-free soft margarine

170g/¾ cup unrefined golden caster (superfine) sugar

100g/3½oz packet ground almonds

3 large organic free-range eggs

A few drops of pure almond extract

3 tablespoons organic milk or dairy-free organic unsweetened soya milk

55g/2 x 1oz squares plain or dairy-free dark chocolate, chopped into small pieces

15g/¼ cup flaked almonds

***coeliacs please use gluten-free ingredients**

Preheat the oven to 170°C/325°F/Gas mark 3.

Sift the flour and baking powder into a large mixing bowl, stir in the margarine, sugar, ground almonds, eggs, almond extract and milk. Using a wooden spoon, beat the mixture for about 1 minute until smooth. Stir in the chocolate pieces.

Spoon the mixture into a standard-sized loaf tin (pan) that has been greased and lined with non-stick baking parchment (wax paper), and level the top. Sprinkle with the flaked almonds and bake for about 1 hour until well risen and golden.

Cool the cake in the tin (pan) and then turn out onto a wire rack to cool completely. Store in an airtight container until needed.

Sticky Prune and Date Cake

You could add some chopped stem ginger to this wonderfully sticky cake and use ginger jam (jelly) instead of apricot jam for a more spicy cake. It keeps for days in an airtight container and is an excellent addition to the work lunchbox if slices are wrapped in baking parchment (wax paper).

Serves 16

GF   V

170g/1 heaped cup whole ready-to-eat pitted prunes, coarsely chopped
225g/1½ cups pitted dates, coarsely chopped
115g/scant cup raisins
115g/scant cup currants
255g/9oz organic butter
400g/14oz can condensed milk
250ml/1 cup cold filtered water
310g/2⅓ cups wheat-free flour mix*
1 teaspoon bicarbonate soda (baking soda)
1 heaped tablespoon warmed apricot jam (jelly) to glaze

20cm/8in square non-stick baking tin (pan), lined with baking parchment (wax paper) or Bake-O-Glide

* coeliacs please use gluten-free ingredients

Preheat the oven to 170°C/325°F/Gas mark 3.

Put all the fruit, butter, condensed milk and water together in a large non-stick pan (it must be non-stick or you may burn the milk) and bring to the boil. Stir frequently to prevent the mixture sticking or burning. Reduce the heat immediately the mixture boils and simmer for 3 minutes. Remove from the heat and leave to cool.

After about 25 minutes, sift the flour and bicarbonate of soda (baking soda) together in a large bowl. Pour the fruit mixture into the flour and mix, using a wooden spoon. Spoon the mixture into the prepared cake tin (pan).

Bake for about 1¼ hours until the cake is firm to the touch. Leave the cake to cool in the tin (pan) and then turn out onto a wire rack. Glaze the top with the warm jam (jelly) and set aside until cold.

Ginger Cake with Ginger Fudge Icing

You can make this cake a couple of days before it is needed and store it, wrapped in clingfilm (plastic wrap), in a cool place. Make the icing on the day of serving or freeze the cake iced.

GF   DF   V

Serves 12–16

Cake

225g/8oz organic butter or dairy-free margarine, diced

170g/1 heaped cup unrefined molasses sugar

3 heaped tablespoons black treacle

150ml/generous ½ cup organic milk or dairy-free organic unsweetened soya milk

2 large organic free-range eggs, beaten

4 balls of stem ginger, drained of their syrup and chopped

300g/1½ cups wheat-free flour mix*

2 teaspoons wheat-free baking powder*

1 tablespoon ground ginger

2 tablespoons ginger syrup from the stem ginger jar

Icing

170g/scant 1½ cups unrefined icing (confectioners') sugar

140g/5oz organic butter or dairy-free margarine

2 tablespoons ginger syrup, from the stem ginger jar

2 teaspoons fresh lemon juice

23cm/9in, deep, loose-bottomed, side-release cake tin (pan), lined with non-stick baking parchment (wax paper) or Bake-O-Glide

coeliacs please use gluten-free ingredients

Preheat the oven to 180°C/350°F/Gas mark 4.

Place the butter or margarine, sugar and treacle in a saucepan and melt over very low heat. Stir, allow to cool for a few minutes and then pour in the milk. Mix and gradually beat the eggs into the melted mixture and then stir in the chopped ginger.

Sift the flour, baking powder and ground ginger together and stir into the mixture. Beat the mixture until smooth. Transfer the cake mixture into the prepared tin (pan) and bake for about 55 minutes. The cake should be firm to touch and have shrunk slightly from the edges. Leave the cake to cool in the tin (pan).

Once the cake has cooled, make some small holes in the top of the cake and drizzle 2 tablespoons of ginger syrup over the cake. When the cake is cold, wrap it in baking parchment (wax paper) and wrap again in kitchen foil and store for 1–2 days.

To make the icing, beat together the icing ingredients until light and smooth. Spread and swirl the icing all over the top of the cake.

Devil's Food Cake

This is a completely over-the-top, utterly sumptuous cake. It can be served for special occasions, teas or as a pudding with vanilla (dairy or dairy-free) ice cream or crème fraîche.

Serves 12–16

GF   DF   V

Cake

155g/5½ × 1oz squares dairy-free dark chocolate* (minimum 72% cocoa solids)

130g/⅔ cup unrefined golden caster (superfine) sugar

125ml/½ cup organic milk or organic dairy-free unsweetened soya milk

55g/½ cup dairy-free cocoa powder

3 large organic free-range eggs, separated, plus 1 extra egg yolk

155g/5½oz softened organic butter or dairy-free margarine

100g/¾ cup unrefined light muscovado sugar

225g/1¾ cups Orgran self-raising gluten-free flour (see page 305 for stockist)

½ teaspoon fine salt

1 heaped teaspoon bicarbonate of soda (baking soda)

250ml/1 cup crème fraîche or Tofutti Sour Supreme sour cream substitute (see page 305 for stockist)

Icing

200g/7 × 1oz squares dairy-free dark chocolate* (73% cocoa solids)

55g/½ cup dairy-free cocoa powder

100ml/scant ½ cup filtered water

1 heaped tablespoon golden (corn) syrup

55g/2oz softened organic butter or dairy-free margarine

225g/1½ cups unrefined icing (confectioners') sugar, sifted

2 large organic free-range egg yolks

2 × 23 cm/9in loose-bottomed, spring-form cake tins (pans), greased and lined with non-stick baking parchment (wax paper) or Bake-O-Glide

* coeliacs please use gluten-free ingredients

Preheat the oven to 180°C/350°F/Gas mark 4.

Put the chocolate, caster (superfine) sugar, milk, cocoa powder and 2 of the egg yolks in a bowl set over simmering water and stir until melted.

Beat the butter or margarine with the muscovado sugar in a food processor until light and fluffy. Beat in the remaining yolks, then the flour, salt and bicarbonate of soda (baking soda). Fold in the crème fraîche or the alternative and then the chocolate mixture.

Whisk the egg whites until stiff and fold them into the cake mixture. Divide the mixture equally between the prepared tins (pan) and bake in the oven for about 40–45 minutes or until a skewer, inserted into the middle of the cake, comes out almost clean. Cool the cakes in the tins (pans) and then turn each one out onto a serving plate, crust side down.

Make the icing. Melt the chocolate in a bowl set over simmering water. In a non-stick pan, melt the cocoa powder, water and syrup until runny. Take the pan off the heat, mix in the chocolate then stir in the butter or margarine, icing (confectioners') sugar and egg yolks until creamy. Cool until spreadable. Beat in a little boiling filtered water if the icing is too thick and sticky.

Cut each sponge in two and sandwich all the sponges together with the icing, keeping enough to spread all over the top and sides of the cake. Leave until cold, cover with clingfilm (plastic wrap) and leave overnight.

Serve at room temperature.

Lemon Almond Cookies

These delicious and crumbly biscuits are sandwiched together with a delicate buttercream. They will keep well in an airtight container for a few days but store them in a cool place because of the buttercream.

Makes 20 filled cookies

GF DF V Q&E

Cookies

255g/9oz organic butter or dairy-free margarine, at room temperature
130g/heaped ½ cup unrefined golden caster (superfine) sugar
2 large organic free-range egg yolks
Finely grated zest of 1 unwaxed lemon
130g/1⅓ cups ground almonds
255g/2⅓ cups wheat-free flour mix*

Lemon buttercream

130g/4½oz organic butter or dairy-free margarine, at room temperature
130g/4½oz unrefined golden caster (superfine) sugar
Finely grated zest of 1 small unwaxed lemon
Finely grated zest of 1 small unwaxed orange

* coeliacs please use gluten-free ingredients

Preheat the oven to 180°C/350°F/Gas mark 4.

Make the cookies first. Beat the butter or margarine with the sugar in a food processor until pale and creamy. Beat in the egg yolks and lemon zest. Briefly mix in the almonds and flour.

Take small lumps of the dough and roll them into 40 small rounds. Put them onto 2 non-stick baking trays and press the prongs of a fork down on each one so that they flatten slightly.

Bake for about 18 minutes, swapping shelves halfway through cooking. The cookies should be tinged with gold but they shouldn't be golden brown. Cool the cookies for 5 minutes before lifting them off the trays and onto wire racks.

To make the filling, beat the butter or margarine with the sugar until soft and fluffy, then mix in the grated lemon and orange rind.

Sandwich the cookies together with the buttercream.

Easy Chocolate Crunch Torte

Everyone has his or her own version of a no-cook chocolate biscuit cake and this is my favourite. If you don't want to use the rum, you can replace it with orange juice or fresh coffee and serve it as a dessert with crème fraîche or dairy-free vanilla ice cream.

GF   DF   V

Serves 12

75g/½ cup dried sour cherries

55g/⅓ cup sultanas (golden raisins)

3 tablespoons rum

225g/8oz dairy-free chocolate* (minimum72% cocoa solids), broken into pieces

55g/2oz organic butter or dairy-free margarine

170g/6oz coarsely broken up amaretti morbidi biscuits (almond macaroons) – make sure alternatives you use are wheat- or gluten-free

55g/½ cup unsalted pistachio nuts, coarsely chopped

200ml/¾ cup organic mascarpone or Provamel dairy-free Soya Dream

Optional

Dairy-free cocoa powder to dust

20.5cm/8in loose-bottomed, non-stick cake tin (pan), lightly greased with flavourless oil or use a standard non-stick loaf tin (pan) lined with clingfilm (plastic wrap)

* coeliacs please use gluten-free ingredients

Soak the cherries and sultanas (golden raisins) in the rum for as long as possible and up to one day in advance.

Melt the chocolate and the butter or margarine in a heatproof bowl over simmering water and stir until glossy. Cool for a few minutes then fold in the marinated fruits, broken up amaretti (almond macaroons), nuts and lastly the mascarpone or Soya Dream.

Spoon the mixture into the prepared cake tin (pan) and smooth over. Chill the torte for about 4 hours. Transfer the torte onto a plate and serve dusted with sieved cocoa.

Baking ...

Raspberry and White Chocolate Muffins

This is a heavenly combination of white chocolate and raspberries. Those who don't like white chocolate – yes there are some – can make these muffins with milk chocolate instead. For a dairy-free version use good quality dark chocolate and dairy-free milk and margarine.

Makes 8

GF   V

285g/2½ cups wheat-free flour mix*, sifted
3 teaspoons wheat-free baking powder*
155g/¾ cup unrefined golden caster (superfine) sugar
2 organic free-range eggs
1 teaspoon pure vanilla extract
225ml/¾ cup organic milk
55g/2oz organic butter, melted
115g/1 cup ripe fresh raspberries or frozen but not defrosted raspberries
85g/3 × 1oz squares El Rey white chocolate (see page 307 for stockist), chopped or other brands*

1 deep muffin tin (pan) lined with 8 large non-stick paper cases

* coeliacs please use gluten-free ingredients

Preheat the oven to 200°C/400°F/Gas mark 6.

Mix the flour and the baking powder in a bowl and stir in the sugar. Briefly whisk the egg, vanilla, milk and melted butter in a separate bowl.

Stir the liquid mixture into the dry ingredients then briefly and gently fold in the raspberries and chocolate. Spoon the mixture into the prepared muffin tin (pan) and bake for about 15 minutes until well risen and only just firm to touch. They will carry on cooking for a minute or two in the tin (pan). Serve the muffins warm so that the chocolate is still gooey.

Rye and Barley Soda Bread

This recipe is for those with a wheat allergy or intolerance – it is not suitable for coeliacs. The great thing about soda bread is that not only is it yeast free but – because of this – it is gloriously quick to make, as there is no rising time. It keeps well for about three days if kept in a sealed polythene bag at room temperature.

V   RF   Q&E

Makes a 455g/1lb loaf

170g/1¼ cups organic rye flour
270g/2 cups organic barley flour
1 heaped tablespoon organic flax seeds
1 heaped teaspoon bicarbonate of soda (baking soda)
½ teaspoon sea salt
30g/1oz organic margarine
1 heaped teaspoon blackstrap molasses
500–600ml/2–2½ cups buttermilk (amount depends on absorbency of flour)

455g/1lb non-stick loaf tin (pan), or a round one if you prefer, greased and floured

Preheat the oven to 220°C/425°F/Gas mark 7.

Place all the dry ingredients in a large bowl and mix them together with your hands, lightly rubbing in the margarine and molasses. Make a well in the centre and add the buttermilk. Working with a metal spoon, from the centre, gather the mixture to make a soft, wet dough. The amount of buttermilk needed will depend on the absorbency of the flour but the mixture should be 'sticky wet'.

Spoon the dough into the prepared tin (pan) and bake for about 35 minutes. Cover the top with foil after 15 minutes. Turn out on to a wire rack and cover with a tea towel. Leave the loaf to cool before attempting to cut it.

Stilton and Poppy Seed Sablés

A good Stilton is an important part of any cheese board, especially at Christmas. A good buying tip is that although the pierced holes may be visible the cheese must not be cracked. Also, do not buy a piece that has been tightly sealed in clingfilm (plastic wrap), as it will be sweaty and salty.

This pastry can be thickly sliced, topped with Stilton and frozen. Cook them from frozen and they will keep in an airtight container for 2–3 days.

Makes about 20

GF   V   Q&E

Sablés
100g/1 cup wheat-free flour mix*
85g/3oz cold organic butter, diced
A small pinch of dried chopped sage leaves
A small pinch of cayenne pepper
1 tablespoon polenta
1 tablespoon poppy seeds
115g/4oz organic Stilton, crumbled
Sea salt and freshly ground black pepper

Extra Stilton to top the sablés

* coeliacs please use gluten-free ingredients

Preheat the oven to 200°C/400°F/Gas mark 6.

Mix the ingredients for the sablés in a food processor until the mixture forms pastry dough. Knead the dough briefly on a floured surface using your hands then roll it out into a sausage shape about 25.5cm/10in long. Wrap the pastry in clingfilm (plastic wrap) and chill for 30 minutes or up to 2 days.

Slice the pastry dough into rounds just under 1cm/½ in thick – unless you are freezing them, in which case they need to be slightly thicker. Lay the sablés on baking sheets with enough room to spread during baking. Place a small piece of Stilton on top of each one and bake for about 10 minutes until the edges are golden and the cheese is bubbling.

Leave the sablés to cool for a couple of minutes before removing them from the baking sheet onto a wire rack. Allow them to cool a little more before serving.

The Big Book of Wheat-Free Cooking

Walnut Bread

Walnut bread is a hearty and delicious accompaniment to soup, pâtés or cheeses. This recipe is not suitable for coeliacs, as it features rye and oats, both of which contain gluten. You will need a bread-making machine for this recipe. You can substitute raisins or sultanas (golden raisins) for the walnuts and you can add seeds or spices.

V   RF

Make 1 extra large loaf

7g/¼oz wheat-free fast-acting yeast
300g/3 cups organic rye flour
300g/3 cups organic oat flour or very fine oatmeal
1½ tablespoons unrefined golden caster (superfine) sugar
2 tablespoons skimmed milk powder
1½ teaspoons sea salt
½ teaspoon vitamin C powder
30g/1oz organic butter
100g/3½oz packet walnut halves
420ml/1¾ cups cold filtered water

Remove the bread pan from the unit. Place the yeast inside the clean pan followed by the flours and the dry ingredients but leave the walnuts until later.

Dot the dry mixture with the butter or margarine, sprinkle with walnuts and pour the water over. Return the pan to the unit, secure as usual and close the lid.

Select the whole-wheat rapid bake option of 3 hours, extra large loaf and dark crust option if possible. Let the bread cool completely on a wire rack. Slice the bread when cold.

Olive and Rosemary Bread

This recipe uses a bread-making machine but you can use it as a guide if you wish to make the loaf by hand. I only ever use a bread-making machine as I never seem to have time for all the pounding and kneading. You can use green olives instead of black if you prefer and other herbs, such as sage or oregano, instead of the rosemary. This bread is delicious with soup, salads or cheeses.

V   RF

Makes 1 extra large loaf

7g/¼oz wheat-free fast-acting yeast
500g/3⅓ cups organic rye flour
55g/¾ cup organic millet flour
55g/¾ cup organic quinoa flour
1½ tablespoons unrefined golden granulated sugar
2 generous tablespoons skimmed milk powder
1½ teaspoons sea salt
1 heaped teaspoon vitamin C powder
2 heaped teaspoons dried finely chopped rosemary
100g/3½oz packet whole pitted black olives, halved
30g/1oz organic butter
420ml/scant 1¾ cups cold filtered water

Remove the bread pan from the unit. Place the yeast inside the clean pan, followed by the flours, the dry ingredients, rosemary and olives.

Dot the dry mixture with the butter and pour the water over, return the pan to the unit, secure as usual and close the lid. Select the whole-wheat, rapid bake option of 3 hours, extra large loaf.

Because the dough is so heavy, it is a good idea to check it after about 30 minutes or whenever the bread is not being kneaded. Use a narrow spatula to scrape any flour or sticky bits of dough away from the sides and the corners, especially at the bottom of the pan. Repeat if necessary.

Leave the bread in the bread maker for about 30 minutes to let the steam soften the crust, turn out the bread and cool completely on a wire rack. It must be cold before slicing.

Mini Rosemary and Orange Muffins

These muffins are great for picnics, buffets and lunch boxes or simply served with soup and cheese.

GF   V   Q&E

Makes 24 mini muffins

55g/2oz organic butter, softened

85g/scant ½ cup unrefined golden caster (superfine) sugar

I large organic free-range egg, beaten

155g/1½ cups wheat-free flour mix*, sifted together with I teaspoon bicarbonate of soda (baking soda) and a good pinch of fine salt

200ml/¾ cup buttermilk

55g/⅓ cup sultanas (golden raisins)

Finely grated rind of I unwaxed orange

I tablespoon freshly chopped rosemary

55g/½ cup chopped walnuts

2 mini muffin trays lined with 24 non-stick mini muffin paper cases

* coeliacs please use gluten-free ingredients

Preheat the oven to 200°C/400°F/Gas mark 6.

Put the butter and sugar into a bowl and cream them together until pale and fluffy. Add the egg, some of the flour, bicarbonate of soda (baking soda) and salt mixture. Fold in the buttermilk, followed by the remaining flour mixture. Add the sultanas (golden raisins), finely grated orange rind, rosemary and walnuts and fold into the mixture.

Spoon the muffin mixture into the paper cases and bake for about 20 minutes until golden and firm. Cool a little on a wire rack and eat warm or store in an airtight container for a couple of days.

Cheese and Chive Scones

For these scones you can use any leftover bits of cheese – the stronger the better – and you can mix different kinds of cheese together for interesting textures and flavours. Goat or sheep cheeses can be used and you can change the herbs to suit the season and the cheese.

Makes 6	GF V Q&E

170g/6oz Orgran wheat-free self-raising flour or other brands* sifted, plus a little extra for dusting (see page 305 for stockist)

½ teaspoon pure mustard powder

A pinch of cayenne pepper

½ teaspoon fine salt

30g/1oz organic butter, plus a little extra for greasing

85g/3oz organic mature hard cheese, grated (Cheshire and Cheddar are perfect)

1 tablespoon chopped fresh chives

1 large organic free-range egg

3 heaped tablespoons buttermilk

For the tops

A little organic milk for brushing

30g/1oz organic mature hard cheese, grated (Cheshire and Cheddar are perfect)

Cayenne pepper

5.5cm/2¼in fluted cutter

* coeliacs please use gluten-free ingredients

Preheat the oven to 220°C/425°F/Gas mark 7.

Sift the flour again, holding it a good height from the bowl. Mix in the mustard powder, cayenne and salt and then rub in the butter until you have a mixture that resembles breadcrumbs. Mix in 85g/3oz of cheese and the chives. Beat in the egg with 3 tablespoons of buttermilk and gradually incorporate the mixture into the dry ingredients. You should have a soft, smooth dough. Don't over-work the dough or the scones will be heavy.

Lightly roll the dough out on a floured board to 2.5cm/1in thick or a little more. Using the fluted cutter, cut out 6 scones, re-rolling the dough if necessary. Place the scones on a baking tray, brush the tops with milk, sprinkle with the remaining cheese and lightly dust with cayenne.

Bake for 15 minutes or until risen and golden brown. Allow the scones to cool a little on a wire rack – they are best served still warm.

Scones

For me, scones are wrapped up in childhood memories of seaside holidays in Cornwall. Split and filled with clotted cream and strawberries they were the ultimate teatime treat. Scones, however, can be cut into triangles, iced or filled with nuts, spices or chocolates chips as they are in America. Here is the basic recipe that you can have fun experimenting with.

GF   V   Q&E

Makes about 20 scones

900g/2lbs white wheat-free flour mix*
2 large pinches of fine salt
6 heaped teaspoons wheat-free baking powder*
170g/6oz organic butter, cubed
55g/⅓ cup unrefined golden caster (superfine) sugar
4 organic free-range eggs
About 500ml/2 cups organic milk (varies according to the absorbency of the flour)

To glaze
1 organic free-range egg whisked with a pinch of fine salt
Unrefined golden granulated sugar

6.5cm/2½ in fluted metal pastry cutter

* coeliacs please use gluten-free ingredients

Preheat the oven to 220°C/425°F/Gas mark 7.

Sieve the flour, salt and baking powder into a large bowl. Lightly rub in the butter using your thumbs and fingertips until the mixture resembles coarse breadcrumbs.

Stir in the sugar and make a well in the centre of the mixture.

Whisk the eggs with the milk and stir into the dry ingredients until it becomes a soft dough. Turn the dough out onto a floured board, lightly shape it into a round and gently roll it out to no less than 2.5cm/1in thick. Cut the dough into scones using the cutter.

Brush the scones with the whisked egg and salt, then dip each one in the sugar. Place on a non-stick baking sheet and bake for about 10–15 minutes until golden brown. Cool on a wire rack and eat the same day.

Apricot and Macadamia Nut Flapjacks

You can vary the fruit and nuts in this recipe according to what you have in your store cupboard. Dried apples and hazelnuts are delicious, as are glacé cherries and almonds.

Makes about 30 small flapjacks

255g/9oz organic butter or dairy-free margarine
200g/7 tablespoons golden (corn) syrup
100g/¾ cup unrefined soft brown sugar
255g/2¾ cups organic rolled oats
100g/¾ cup wheat-free flour mix
115g/¾ cup dried apricots, coarsely chopped
100g/3½oz packet macadamia nuts, coarsely chopped

34cm/12in Swiss roll tin (pan), lined with non-stick baking parchment (wax paper) or Bake-O-Glide

Preheat the oven to 180°C/350°F/Gas mark 4.

Melt the butter or margarine, syrup and sugar together over low heat until melted, stirring occasionally. Put the oats, flour, apricots and nuts into a big bowl and stir in the liquid ingredients until well combined.

Transfer the mixture into the prepared tin (pan) and press down firmly.

Bake in the oven for about 20–25 minutes until golden. Leave the flapjacks to cool in the tin (pan) before cutting into squares and carefully removing to an airtight container.

Rosewater and Cinnamon Mince Pies

Christmas is very special to me. I love the spirit of giving and sharing, the traditional carols, music, feasting and just being with all the family in front of a roaring log fire. The excitement of decorating the Christmas tree on Christmas Eve and the expectant joy of the children waiting for Father Christmas makes the days spent preparing and cooking worthwhile. These mince pies freeze beautifully; defrost them and bake them until they are hot and ready to eat.

Makes 30 mini or 24 standard pies

GF **DF** **V**

Pastry
255g/2¼ cups wheat-free flour mix*

125g/4½oz organic butter or dairy-free margarine, cut into 12 small pieces

Pinch of sea salt

1 large organic free-range egg

A little rosewater (available from superstores or pharmacies)

Filling
255g/1 cup luxury mincemeat for the mini mince pies or 426g/1½ cups for the standard size (vegetarian brands are available at health food stores)

¼ teaspoon ground cinnamon

About ½ tablespoon unrefined golden caster (superfine) sugar mixed with ½ teaspoon ground cinnamon for sprinkling

3 × 12-cup non-stick mini muffin tins (pans) or 2 × 12-cup standard muffin or mince pie non-stick baking tins (pans)

A fluted pastry circle cutter approximately 5cm/2in for the pastry bases and a smaller cutter for the tops in a star shape for the mini pies, and 8cm/3in cutter for the bases and 5cm/2in cutter for the tops of the standard pies

* coeliacs please use gluten-free ingredients

Preheat the oven to 180°C/350°F/Gas mark 4.

Make the pastry in the food processor. Put all the pastry ingredients, except the rosewater, in the processor and whizz for a few seconds until the mixture resembles breadcrumbs. Gradually add the rosewater, processing briefly until it comes together into a ball of dough. Remove the dough, wrap it in clingfilm (plastic wrap) and freeze for 10 minutes.

Mix the sugar and the ½ teaspoon cinnamon together in a little bowl and leave until needed. Roll out the dough on a floured board into a medium–thick pastry and then cut into 24 circles. Line the cups of the baking tin (pan) with the pastry circles and prick the bases with a fork. Gather the remaining pastry, roll it out again with a little more flour and cut out 24 smaller circles for the lids.

In a small bowl, mix the mincemeat with the cinnamon, spoon about a teaspoonful into each pastry case and gently press it down as you cover the mixture with the pastry lid. Sprinkle all the mince pies with the cinnamon and sugar mixture and bake in the centre of the oven for about 15 minutes or until the pastry is golden and the mincemeat bubbling.

Leave them to cool in the tins (pans) and then lift the mince pies out using a blunt knife. Leave them to cool further on wire racks. Warm the mince pies through before serving, or alternatively, freeze in an airtight container until needed.

Lemon Muffins

I love zingy lemon recipes, which this one certainly is! These muffins are great for picnics (top some of them with lemon icing for children) and the leftovers are still delicious for breakfast with fresh fruit and yogurt or yofu, or for lunch with fresh fruit salad. The ingredients can easily be halved to make fewer muffins.

GF   **DF**   **V**   **Q&E**

Makes 18

Muffins

2 tablespoons poppy seeds

2 tablespoons runny honey

2 tablespoons lemon juice, plus finely grated rind and juice of 1 unwaxed lemon

110g/½ cup organic butter or dairy-free margarine

110g/½ cup unrefined golden caster (superfine) sugar

2 large free-range eggs

170ml/scant cup plain live soy yogurt (provamol makes yofu) or a low-fat live goats' or sheeps' yogurt if you are not sensitive to these products

200g/1¾ cups wheat-free flour mix*

2 teaspoons wheat-free baking powder*

1 teaspoon bicarbonate of soda (baking soda)

12-cup muffin tin (pan) and a 6-cup muffin tin (pan) lined with 18 paper cases

---

* coeliacs please use gluten-free ingredients

Preheat the oven to 180°C/350°F/Gas mark 4.

Mix the poppy seeds, honey and 2 tablespoons of lemon juice in a small pan; bring to the boil over a medium heat and cook for a couple of seconds. Cool and stir in the remaining lemon juice and grated rind.

In a food processor, beat together the margarine and sugar until smooth and then briefly mix in the eggs, yogurt and the seed mixture. Very briefly whizz in the flour, baking powder and bicarbonate of soda (baking soda).

Divide the mixture between the muffin cups and bake for about 20 minutes until golden and springy to the touch.

Breakfasts ...

Deluxe Muesli

We eat this delicious muesli often during the warmer months, whilst in winter we opt for porridge. This recipe is not suitable for coeliacs but could easily be adapted by substituting gluten-free grains or flakes for the oats, barley and rye flakes.

Fills a 2 litre/3½ pint plastic container

DF   V   RF   Q&E

100g/1 cup organic porridge oats
130g/1 cup organic millet flakes
100g/1 cup organic barley flakes
130g/1 cup organic rice flakes
100g/1 cup organic rye flakes
100g/1 cup organic quinoa flakes
255g/8oz packet sun-dried apricots, chopped
120g/1 cup chopped walnut pieces or pecan pieces
60g/½ cup sunflower seeds
60g/½ cup pumpkin seeds
1–2 teaspoons ground cinnamon

Mix all the ingredients together, transfer to an airtight container and seal until needed.

Figgy Orange Muffins

Ready-to-eat dried figs are succulently sweet without the 'chewiness' of the firmer dried figs. These figs make delicious spicy muffins for a filling winter breakfast.

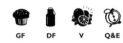

Makes 12

GF   DF   V   Q&E

225g/8oz wheat-free flour mix*
1 tablespoon wheat-free baking powder*
½ teaspoon bicarbonate of soda (baking soda)
75g/⅓ cup unrefined demerara sugar
1 teaspoon ground cinnamon
Finely grated rind of 1 unwaxed orange
150ml/generous ½ cup organic milk or organic unsweetened dairy-free soya milk
2 organic free-range eggs
55g/2oz organic butter or dairy-free margarine, melted
255g/9oz pack ready-to-eat figs, stalks removed, finely chopped

Topping
1 teaspoon unrefined demerara sugar
½ teaspoon ground cinnamon

12-cup, non-stick, deep muffin tin (pan) lined with circles of baking parchment (wax paper) or Bake-O-Glide

* coeliacs please use gluten-free ingredients

Preheat the oven to 200°C/400°F/Gas mark 6.

In a large bowl, mix the flour, baking powder, bicarbonate of soda (baking soda), sugar, cinnamon and the finely grated orange rind. In a jug, mix the milk, eggs and melted butter or margarine and then pour it over the dry ingredients. Briefly fold the ingredients together using a metal spoon and then gently fold in the figs.

Spoon the mixture into the prepared muffin tin (pan). Make the topping by mixing the sugar and cinnamon. Sprinkle the mixture over the muffins and bake for about 15 minutes until risen and just firm. Cool slightly, transfer to a wire rack and serve warm.

Muesli Breakfast Muffins

These are great muffins for munching at breakfast and definitely worth getting out of bed for.

Makes 12

GF   V   Q&E

115g/4oz ready-to-eat dried apricots, chopped
4 tablespoons fresh orange juice
2 large organic free-range eggs
200ml/¾ cup buttermilk
100ml/⅓ cup cold pressed sunflower oil
85g/scant ½ cup unrefined golden caster (superfine) sugar
300g/2¾ cups wheat-free flour mix*
3 teaspoons wheat-free baking powder*
55g/½ cup wheat-free muesli mix*
12 teaspoons marmalade

Topping
55g/generous ½ cup unrefined light muscovado sugar
2 tablespoons cold pressed sunflower oil
55g/generous ½ cup wheat-free muesli*

2 × 6-bun muffin tins (pans), lined with paper cases

coeliacs please use gluten-free ingredients

Preheat the oven to 200°C/400°F/Gas mark 6.

Put the apricots and orange juice in a medium bowl and leave to soak for about half an hour to plump the apricots up. In another bowl, beat the eggs with the buttermilk, oil and sugar. Stir the mixture into the apricots. In a large bowl, combine the flour, baking powder and muesli and then gently stir in the apricot mixture. Mix gently and quickly and turn the mixture into the muffin tin (pan).

Coat the tip of your thumb with some flour and quickly make a deep thumbprint in the centre of each muffin. Fill each indentation with a teaspoon of marmalade. Combine the topping ingredients, sprinkle them over the top of each muffin and bake for about 20 minutes until well risen and golden.

Cool the muffins slightly in the tin (pan) and then on wire racks for about 10 minutes before eating them warm and fresh.

American Pancakes

You can quickly make a stack of these fluffy, American-style pancakes for breakfast to keep the family fuelled for the morning. If you are a late starter, simply enjoy them for brunch!

Serves 4   GF   DF   V   Q&E

255g/2½ cups wheat-free flour mix*
3 heaped teaspoons wheat-free baking powder*
1 teaspoon sea salt
3 tablespoons unrefined golden caster (superfine) sugar
250ml/1 cup organic milk or organic unsweetened soya milk
2 organic free-range eggs, lightly beaten
55g/2oz organic butter or dairy-free margarine, melted, plus extra for cooking
Maple syrup and a knob of organic butter or dairy-free margarine to serve

***coeliacs please use alternative ingredients**

Sift the flour, baking powder, salt and sugar into a bowl. In another bowl, mix the milk, eggs and melted butter or margarine then stir into the dry ingredients. Transfer the mixture to a large jug.

Heat a little butter or margarine in a non-stick frying pan (skillet) over medium heat, pour in spoonfuls of the batter and cook the pancakes in batches until all the batter is used up. Cook each pancake for about 1–2 minutes on one side and when bubbles form on top of the pancake and the underside is golden, flip it over and cook the other side for 1 minute. Keep the pancakes warm while you cook the remaining batches.

Meanwhile, heat the maple syrup together with the butter or margarine and serve warm with the pancakes.

Blender Fruit Smoothie

Fruit smoothies provide the perfect cocktail of vitamins and energy to start the day. You can use any seasonal fruits and, if you experiment with your favourite fruits, you will invent some gorgeous blends. You will soon have special textures and flavours that you like for different moods. Here are my two favourite combinations for summer.

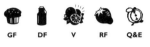

Serves 1

GF   DF   V   RF   Q&E

Option 1
1 sweet apple, peeled, quartered, cored and sliced
Juice of ½ a lime
150g/1 cup fresh, ripe raspberries
1 ripe, peeled and stoned (pitted) peach, coarsely chopped

Option 2
1 ripe, peeled and stoned (pitted) nectarine, coarsely chopped
Juice of ½ a small lemon
100g/1 cup ripe, freshly chopped pineapple flesh
1 sweet and ripe pear, peeled, quartered and core removed

Process all the ingredients for your chosen option in a blender until smooth. Pour into a glass and drink immediately.

Menu Planning Tips

Some of my friends tell me that the bit they hate most about giving a party is the menu planning. Personally, I think it's the best bit! I can spend hours drooling over glorious food pictures in glossy magazines and cookbooks, usually putting together such a stunning menu that it would take me about three days to prepare it. Inevitably, I then lose the plot and make something I have made a hundred times before! To prevent this happening to you I have given some useful guidelines below. This is followed by a selection of seasonal menus that you can mix and match with the remaining recipes in the book. They are included merely as guides and are useful if you don't want to spend hours reading through the recipes every time you want to entertain. You will also find an index of recipes on page 299 – this will make it easier for you to plan your own menus as it allows you to see all the recipes at a glance.

Guidelines

- Choose your main course first, then the first course and finally, the dessert to complement.
- The first course should be light enough to whet the palate, set the mood for the rest of the meal and not make you so full that you struggle through the next course.
- Consider the occasion when you decide on your menu. You don't want to go over the top for an informal kitchen supper or your guests may be embarrassed; neither do you want to prepare an obviously quick and easy menu as your guests may think that you haven't made any effort at all for them.
- Decide on the most likely tastes of your guests so that you don't give them exotic food when they love plain and simple food or vice versa. I think it's polite to ask any guests that you do not know well if there is any food that they do not eat. By this I am not referring to any faddish preferences they may have, rather if they are, for example, vegetarian or have a food intolerance. It is usually possible for them to pick out the unwanted ingredient in a salad, for example, or you can bake a chicken breast without the mushroom sauce if

mushrooms are unacceptable. Anyone who has an allergy to shellfish, nuts, eggs or other ingredients or is a coeliac will almost certainly warn you in advance.

- Think about the season and the weather; you don't want to serve a hot soup, stew and steamed pudding in summer! Nor do you want to serve chilled soup, salad and ice cream in winter. If it is a cold and wet summer's day you can balance a hot, seasonal soup with a light fish dish and follow with an indulgent, comforting pudding. People can generally digest heartier meals in winter when we often need warming and comforting food. In summer, people generally prefer lighter Mediterranean-style dishes that are refreshing, cooling and easy to digest.

- Choose ingredients that are in season so that they are full of flavour and sweetness and, hopefully, marginally cheaper.

- Unless you don't have to worry about costs, make sure that the menu fits your budget. There is nothing more unsettling than getting half way through the shopping list and then panicking over the unexpected expense. You can juggle menus around so that, for example, you have a cheap soup balanced with an expensive fish dish, followed by a not-too-extravagant pudding. It also helps if you buy fruit and vegetables when there is a glut, or game when it is getting towards the end of the season. Pheasant, for instance, is often half its usual price by the end of January, when the farms and estates have more than they can cope with.

- The number of dishes you serve also needs to be considered. Don't make so many that you spend all evening carrying food around to everyone. If you have a small kitchen or dining area, limit the dishes to two for the main course. A good example is to serve a beef casserole in its dish and a bowl of rice mixed with the vegetables – not roasts with gravy, trimmings, vegetables and stuffing!

- If you are entertaining single-handed, or with little help, plan the menu so that as much as possible is made in advance – even the potatoes or rice can be cooked in advance and kept warm. Otherwise, 'semi' prepare dishes for a quick flourish of activity at the last minute.

- Remember to balance the menu – use contrasting but not conflicting tastes. Don't have a carrot and orange soup followed by chicken and carrots and marmalade ice cream for dessert. Check that the colour scheme is not repetitive too – you don't want to serve green pea soup followed by a green Thai curry. If you have included various vegetables in a casserole, it's a good idea not to serve the same ones as an accompaniment; instead use contrasting vegetables.

- Lastly, use different cooking methods throughout the meal. Don't serve fried squid followed by fried steak and apple fritters. Instead, follow the fried squid with a baked fish or chicken dish and a simple, refreshing pudding.

With all these tips for menu planning you should find putting together a balanced and fun menu easy and relaxing, which should of course make your meal even more enjoyable.

The Big Book of Wheat-Free Cooking

Useful Tips for the Kitchen

- Keep knives sharp – sharp knives are safer than blunt knives
- Never leave a sharp knife in the sink or washing up bowl
- Don't wash your sharp knives in the dishwasher
- Turn the handles of saucepans inwards on the cooker
- Change tea towels and washing up cloths regularly to avoid cross contamination
- Ensure that both the refrigerator and deep-freeze are working at the correct temperature
- Food should be in perfect condition before it is frozen
- Don't put any warm food in the refrigerator or deep-freeze in case other food deteriorates
- Egg whites freeze well (30g = 1 egg white when using them later)
- Hard cheeses, Camembert, Brie and blue-veined cheeses freeze well, in pieces, grated or whole for tarts, pies, pasta dishes and wheat-free toasted sandwiches
- Cream can be frozen if whipped
- Soft fruits freeze well for mousses, pies, sauces and ices
- Tomatoes freeze well for stews, sauces and soups
- Wrap freezer food up properly or it will get freezer burn
- For convenience, freeze small quantities of chicken or vegetable stock (bouillon) to use in recipes
- Slice your wheat-free breads and wrap them individually for easy use in recipes

Menu Plans

Autumn and Winter

Christmas Eve for 8

Parmesan Biscuits with Smoked Salmon and
  Crème Fraîche
Italian Roast Partridge
A selection of vegetables*
Cranberry Trifle

Christmas Day

Roast turkey* with Sage and Hazelnut Stuffing
(vegetarian option – Roast Vegetable,
  Chestnut and Polenta Tarts)
Creamy Bread Sauce
Traditional trimmings, sauces, gravy and
  vegetables*
Christmas pudding* (see page 304 for stockist)
  and Foolproof Boozy Custard
Rosewater and Cinnamon Mince Pies

New Year's Eve for 12

Mini Potato Pancakes with Smoked Trout and
  Salsa
Beef Casserole with Dijon Croûtons
A selection of vegetables*
Devil's Food Cake served with crème fraîche

Boxing Day Leftovers Dinner for 6–8

Fennel and Parsnip Soup
Buckwheat Galettes with Ham and Cheese
Mixed continental salad*
Christmas Mincemeat Torte

Vegetarian Dinner for 6–8

Carrot and Swede Soup
Olive and Rosemary Bread
Mushroom and Garlic Roulade
Mixed roast vegetables*
Lemon Cheesecake

* Recipes not in this book

Sunday Lunch for 6

Traditional Lasagne
Mixed fresh salad*
Spiced Bread Pudding

Cheap and Easy for 4

Stuffed Mushrooms
Fettuccini with Rocket Pesto
Mixed leaf and herb salad*
Apple and Lemon Streusel Cake

Fishy for 4

Katie's Parsnips – place on a bed of rocket salad
    and sunblush tomatoes and serve with
    crème fraîche
Thai Seafood Casserole
Thai fragrant rice*
Key Lime Pie

Weekend Dinner for 6

Spinach, Mushroom and Garlic Croûton Salad
Braised Spiced Lamb Shanks
Mashed celeriac and winter vegetables*
Individual Queen of Puddings

Spring and Summer

Alfresco Lunch for 8

Roasted Vegetable and Goats' Cheese Salad
Chicken, Broad Bean and Bacon Salad
New potatoes*
Baked Alaska

Celebration Dinner for 4

Wrapped Asparagus with Quick Hollandaise
    Sauce
Salmon and Watercress en Croûte
New potatoes and mixed salad*
Honey, Almond and Thyme Ice Cream served
    with florentines* or amaretti (almond)
    biscuits*

Vegetarian Dinner al Fresco for 4

Chickpea, Avocado and Sweet Pepper Salad
Walnut Bread
Torta di Risotto
Mixed green and herb salad*
Peach and Amaretti Tart

Picnic in the Park for 6

Green and Yellow Wax Bean Salad
Summer Mexican Beef Wraps
Puy Lentil Salad
Mixed green and herb salad*
Raspberry and White Chocolate Muffins
Porter Cake

Cheap and Easy for 4–6

Piedmontese Peppers
Pastitsio
Mixed Continental leaf salad and fresh herbs*
Gooseberry Sauce Cake

Sunday Lunch for 8

Chicken with Olives and Potatoes
Mixed roasted summer vegetables*
Chocolate Almond Gâteau
Fresh strawberries and raspberries*

* Recipes not in this book

Vegetarian Dinner for 6

Crème Fraîche and Sundried Tomato Penne
Broccoli and Blue Cheese Tart
Mixed green salad with herbs*
Muscovado Meringues with Lime Cream

All-in-Advance Dinner for 4

Smoked Salmon and Crab Timbales
Rye and Barley Soda bread
Steak with Parmesan and Mushrooms
A selection of steamed green vegetables*
New potatoes*
Raspberry and Pecan Roulade

Weekend Dinner for 6

Caesar Salad with Parmesan Crisps
Pork Braised with Fennel and Artichoke
    Hearts
Potatoes, either mashed or Dauphinoise*
Blackberry Meringue Chill

Reduced Fat Menus
for Summer

Simple and Delicious for 8

Summer Cooler Soup
Penne with Trout, Fresh Peas and Lemon
Large mixed salad*
Peach Angel Ring with Strawberry Coulis

Vegetarian Dinner for 4

Asparagus Salad with Coriander and Ginger
    Dressing
Vegetable Spring Rolls
Fresh spinach*
Raspberry and Pecan Roulade

Reduced Fat Menus
for Winter

Weekend Dinner for 4

Artichoke Chowder
Chicken with Rosemary and Verjuice
Steamed vegetables*
Passion Cakes with Passion Fruit Sauce

Weekend Lunch for 4

Artichoke, Butter Bean and Fennel Salad
Mushroom and Mozzarella Lasagne
Large mixed salad*
Baked Apples with Spiced Cranberry Stuffing

* Recipes not in this book

Index of Recipes

Fish and Seafood

Meat, Poultry and Game

Salads

Vegetarian Main Courses

Vegetables and Accompaniments

Useful Information and Addresses

Antoinette Savill has a website with news, helpful hints and recipes for those with a sensitivity to wheat. The site also includes details of her other books, a credit card hotline for purchasing books from Harper Collins publishers, and her range of gluten- or wheat-free products from Wellfoods Ltd. Website: www.allergywatchers.com

Antoinette has a range of delicious, freshly-baked, gluten-, wheat- and dairy-free foods – The Antoinette Savill Signature Series, which is available from Waitrose, Budgens, The Co-op and other stores and health food shops throughout the UK. The range is also available by mail order from Wellfoods Ltd. Contact details are listed on page 304.

Organizations

Useful information and help can be obtained from the following organizations.

Institute for Optimum Nutrition
Blades Court
Deodar Road
London
SW15 2NU
Telephone: 020 8877 9993

The Coeliac Society
PO Box 220
High Wycombe
Buckinghamshire
HP 11 2HY
Telephone: 01494 437278

Berrydales Publishers
Berrydale House
5 Lawn Road
London
NW3 2XS
Telephone: 020 7722 2866
(Publishers of *The Inside Story* food and health magazine)

British Allergy Foundation
30 Bellegrove Road
Welling
Kent
DA 16 3PY
Telephone: 020 8303 8525

Stockists

This is my list of the best or most appropriate ingredients and stockists that I used throughout this book. I have spent years testing many different brands and the most successful ingredients have only been specified in the recipes if the outcome made a substantial difference to the results.

Wellfoods Ltd (Antoinette Savill food range)
A nationwide delivery of gluten-free and wheat-free flour, white loaves, bread rolls and pizza bases and cakes that can be frozen. The bread should be sliced and then frozen in one pack or individually. The rolls should be baked until soft and hot and the pizza can be frozen in quarters or whole for hungry teenagers! The muffins can be served with vanilla ice cream or used as part of a chocolate trifle.
Telephone: 01226 381712
Fax: 01226 381858
Website: www.bake-it.com
Email: wellfoods@bake-it.com

The Village Bakery (organic breads and cakes)
These are my favourite organic wheat-free brown rye breads, especially the one with raisins (Baltic Rye and Borodinsky Raisin). They also produce a fabulous organic wheat- and gluten-free chocolate almond cake, which serves 16 – I keep one in the deep-freeze for chaotic weekends when friends and family are staying. Their lemon cake is the sponge I use in my trifles and Baked Alaska and they have a huge selection of cakes, flapjacks and Christmas goodies – including Christmas cake. They also run baking courses in Cumbria.
Telephone: 01768 881515
Fax: 01768 881848
Website: www.village-bakery.com
Email: info@village-bakery.com

Provamel Alpro (UK) Ltd (milks)
This is my favourite soya milk – I think that it has the nicest taste, colour and consistency. It is also low in fat and is made from non-GMO soya beans. I used their milks, cream (soya dream), yogurts and desserts throughout this book and they definitely gave the best results. The great news is that many of their products are now organic. Two great ideas: try the vanilla milk hot for a soothing winter cup of coffee that doesn't curdle! In summer, use the Yofu yogurts in your ice cream maker combined with some fresh berries for instant frozen yogurt puddings.
Telephone: 01536 720605
Fax: 01536 725793
Website: www.provamel.co.uk
Email: commercialUK@alpro.be

Tofutti UK Ltd (cheeses)
The best range of cream-style cheese dips that
I tasted; called Creamy Smooth, they come in
3 different flavours. They are not only great in
the recipes but also perfect for spreading on
crispbreads. For making a cheesecake, use the
excellent Sour Supreme sour cream substitute.
They also have a delicious range of ice creams
that can be used to fill Pavlovas or roulades or
served with sauce or fruits. All products,
according to Tofutti Ltd, are yeast-free, GMO-
free, lactose-free, vegetarian, vegan and kosher.
Telephone: 020 8861 4443
Fax: 020 8861 0444
Website: www.tofutti.co.uk

The Redwood Wholefood Company (cheeses)
Dairy- and lactose-free Cheezly cheeses such as
Feta-style in oil is brilliant for pizzas, pasta,
risotto and salads; the grated Cheddar-style
Cheezly hard cheese is the best alternative that
I have found and is used in lots of the recipes.
You can buy them at the on-line shop or at any
good health shop.
Telephone: 01536 400 557
Fax: 01536 408 878
Website: www.redwoodfoods.co.uk
Email: info@redwoodfoods.co.uk

Orgran Community Foods Ltd (pasta, self-raising
flour and breadcrumbs)
Stockists of the gluten-, wheat- and yeast-free
pasta that I use in most of the recipes,
especially the organic rice and corn pasta and
lasagne. If you don't have time to make you
own breadcrumbs use their excellent
breadcrumbs instead. Their pastas include:
fettuccini, tortelli, spaghetti, farfalle (bows),
penne (quills), rigatone (tubes), conchiglie
(shells), lasagne and others. The self-raising
flour is fabulous as part of pastry recipes or for
cakes.
Telephone: 020 8208 2966
Fax: 020 8208 1551
Email: sales@communityfoods.co.uk
Website: www.communityfoods.co.uk

Doves Farm Foods
I use their buckwheat, rye, gluten-free and rice
flour in recipes in this book. The rye is organic,
which particularly appeals to me. They offer
nationwide delivery of all the wheat-free and
gluten-free flours if you can't get them in your
local stores. They also have delicious organic
gluten-free Lemon Zest Cookies, which I use
for cheesecakes.
Telephone: 01488 684 880
Website: www.dovesfarm.co.uk

Allergycare (chocolates)
Brilliant Whizzers dairy-, gluten-, yeast- and
wheat-free speckled eggs, chocolate beans,
chocolate footballs and other sweeties. They
also stock gluten- and yeast-free baking powder
and egg replacer.
Telephone: 01491 570000
Website: www.gfdiet.com

D & D Chocolates (carob and chocolate)
A very good range of mail order gluten-, wheat-, yeast-, dairy-, sugar-free Christmas chocolates and carob such as Father Christmas and snowmen. In addition, Easter eggs, mini eggs plus everyday goodies such as pralines, couverture bars and peppermint creams. Allergy-free carob flakes and chocolate drops (chips) are also available. They are ideal for decorating cakes, making recipes or as lovely gifts.
Telephone 01509 216400
Fax: 01509 233961
Website: www.d-dchocolates.com

www.Allergyfreedirect.co.uk (dairy-free Parmesan)
This is a brilliant site for ordering most things that you will need on any of the usual diets: dairy-free Parmesan (Florentino Parmazano), flours, grains and pulses, cereals and baking ingredients are all available. Their 24-hour courier service is expensive so it's best to go through the site and order anything you may need for the next few months.
Telephone: 01865 722 003
Fax: 01865 244 134
Email: orders@allergyfreedirect.co.uk

Essential Dressings Ltd (Flavoured oils)
This is the source of the amazing little bottles of flavoured oils that I use in the recipes. I have only used three so far – lavender, thyme and ginger – but they have lots of amazing herb and spice flavoured oils. As you only use a few drops, they last for a couple of years, which makes them a very good investment.
Telephone and Fax: 01684 575954
Email: kevinchef@tinyworld.co.uk

Simply Organic Food Company
They stock everything organic – fruit, vegetables, fish, poultry, meat, as well as groceries, baby food, wines and wheat- or lactose-free products. All can be delivered to your home or office throughout the UK. Open 24 hours a day, seven days a week.
Telephone: 0845 1000 444
Fax: 020 7622 4447
Website: www.simplyorganic.net
Email: orders@simplyorganic.net

Sel de Guerande
This sea salt is hand-harvested in the Guerande salt marshes and dried by the sun and wind so that it retains all the magnesium, salts and trace elements.
Telephone: 02 40 62 01 25
Fax: 02 40 62 03 93
Email: lsg@seldeguerande.com

Musk's
Makers of sausages since 1884, they produce gluten-free sausages of various sizes. They now have a mail order service with overnight courier – ideal for Christmas hampers and parties all year round.
Telephone: 01638 662626
Email: office@musks.com

Bake-O-Glide
This is an amazing extra thick, reusable, easy to clean, non-stick liner. It doesn't crinkle and I use it to roll out pastry or cookies on, especially when making gluten-free recipes. It comes in rolls, sheets and pre-cut circles for different standard-sized cake tins.
Telephone: 01706 224790
Website: www.bake-o-glide.co.uk
Email: info@bake-o-glide.co.uk

El Rey Chocolate

This excellent chocolate is available from good delicatessens, Waitrose and specialist confectioners in the UK. They use only 100% Venezuelan Cacao and the 73.5% Apamate is extra-bitter with a smooth and prolonged cacao taste. This will make exceptional chocolate cake, biscuits, ice cream and gâteaux.
Telephone: 020 7854 7770
Website: www.elrey.co.uk
Email: info@elrey.co.uk

Artisan Bread Ltd

This company sells organic, yeast-free, salt-free, high-fibre bread that uses stone ground rye and is baked with pure spring water. It stays fresh for about a week, freezes well and makes you feel really healthy.
Telephone: 01227 771881
Fax: 01227 278661
Email: mail@artisanbread.ltd.uk
Website: www.artisanbread.ltd.uk

Nutrition Point Ltd

Makers of Dietary Specials range of breads and rolls.
Telephone: 01925 258000
Fax: 01925 258001
Email: info@nutritionpoint.co.uk

Index

porter cake 257
potato pancakes with smoked trout 42–3
prawn
  mango and cucumber salad 150
  spicy poppadums 46
  tostaditas with guacamole 89
preservatives 3, 8, 20
processed foods 1
prune, almond and cognac tart 244–5
pumpkin
  pie 246–7
  soup 28–9
puy lentil salad 135

queen of puddings 242–3
quinoa
  couscous 108–9
  risotto 167

rack of lamb with courgettes and broad beans 120
raspberry
  and pecan roulade 228–9
  and white chocolate muffins 270
refrigerator ingredients 16
restaurants 7
rhubarb and oatmeal possets 226
roast dishes
  cod with pineapple salsa 84–5
  halibut with rosemary 70
  Italian partridge 98–9
  skate with baby vegetables 58–9
roasted vegetables
  chestnut and polenta tarts 152–3
  and goats' cheese salad 136
rocket pesto 157
rosemary
  monkfish and pancetta kebabs 62
  and orange muffins 275
rosewater and cinnamon mince pies 280–1
rye and barley soda bread 271

sage and hazelnut stuffing 193
salmon
  fingers with sugar snap salad 148–9
  and lime salad 128
  and watercress en croûte 64–5
sardines with pine nuts and spinach 71

scallops with pak choi 76–7
scones 276–8
seafood casserole 63
seasonal foods 8, 20
sesame salmon fingers 148–9
skate with baby summer vegetables 58–9
smoked salmon
  and crab timbales 44–5
  oriental 87
soy sauce 1, 6–7
spaghetti with ham and flageolet bean sauce 97
spelt 4
spicy dishes
  bread pudding 240–1
  prawn poppadums 46
  squash quarters 199
  tuna on noodles 78–9
spinach
  and lemon risotto 175
  mushroom and garlic croûton salad 139
squash quarters 199
squid
  in breadcrumbs 66
  with herb dressing 80–1
steak with Parmesan and mushrooms 94–5
sticky prune and date cake 261
Stilton and poppy seed sablés 272
store cupboard ingredients 15–16
strawberry coulis 230–1
stuffed dishes
  mushrooms 49
  sardines with pine nuts 71
substitutes 8
sugar snap salad 148–9
summer dishes
  cooler soup 30
  Mexican beef wraps 116–17
  mixed salad 143
  pilaf with hummus 138
summer mixed salad 143
super cheat dishes
  fish pie 61
  orange creams 208
supermarkets 3
sweet potatoes
  griddled 174
  wedges 198
sweet red pepper dip 56

swordfish Palermo 86

tagliatelle with dolcelatte and walnut sauce 158
ten-minute chocolate puddings 238
tests 4, 5
Thai dishes
  fish cakes 74–5
  seafood casserole 63
  winter stir-fry 171
three-bean salad 174
tomatoes
  and olive compote 122–3
  and pesto tarts 50–1
torta di risotto 162–3
tortelli with tuna, lemon and caper sauce 68
tostaditas
  with crab and mango 90
  with guacamole and prawns 89
  with sweetcorn and pepper 90
traditional lasagne 104–5
trout
  and guacamole rolls 73
  in oatmeal 60
tuna on noodles 78–9

vegetables
  barbecued 197–200
  cheese and onion pie 164–5
  kebabs 144–5
  spring rolls 52–3
vitamins 3

walnut
  bread 273
  and rice salad 144–5
warm bread, bacon and poached egg salad 133
water 9
wax bean salad 137
weight loss 2
Welsh rarebit 48
wheat-containing foods 11–12
wild mushroom tortelli 166
winter Thai stir-fry 171
withdrawal symptoms 4
wrapped asparagus with hollandaise sauce 54

yogurt dip 144–5

Index
311

Make
www.thorsonselement.com
your online sanctuary

Get online information, inspiration and
guidance to help you on the path to physical
and spiritual well-being. Drawing on the integrity
and vision of our authors and titles, and with
health advice, articles, astrology, tarot, a
meditation zone, author interviews and events
listings, www.thorsonselement.com is a great
alternative to help create space and peace
in our lives.

So if you've always wondered about practising
yoga, following an allergy-free diet, using the
tarot or getting a life coach, we can point you
in the right direction.

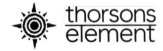

thorsons
element